Fina... ...
Multiple Choice Questions

KT-430-803

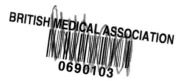

Final FRCA:
Multiple Choice Questions

Michael D Brunner, MBBS FRCA
Consultant Anaesthetist,
Northwick Park and St Mark's Hospitals,
Harrow, UK

P Neville Robinson, MBCh FRCA
Consultant Anaesthetist,
Northwick Park and St Mark's Hospitals,
Harrow, UK

Huw Williams, MBBS FRCA
Specialist Registrar in Anaesthesia,
St Thomas's Hospital, London, UK

BUTTERWORTH
HEINEMANN

EDINBURGH LONDON NEW YORK OXFORD PHILADELPHIA
ST LOUIS SYDNEY TORONTO 2000

Butterworth-Heinemann
Robert Stevenson House, 1-3 Baxter's Place, Leith Walk
Edinburgh EH1 3AP

First published 2000
Reprinted 2004

British Library Cataloguing in Publication Data
Brunner, Michael D.
    Final FRCA: multiple choice questions
    1. Anesthesiology – Examinations, questions, etc.
    I. Title   II. Robinson, P. Neville   III.   William, Huw
    617.9'6'076

ISBN 0 7506 4214 9

Printed and bound in Great Britain by Biddles Ltd,
King's Lynn, Norfolk

Contents

Preface

The final FRCA examination cannot be undertaken without study. Appropriate knowledge must be acquired. The syllabus is enormous and eclectic. A candidate must prepare by practising for the vivas, short answers and the multiple choice questions.

These multiple choice questions have been designed to test and educate. The questions have been chosen carefully having read the Royal College of Anaesthetists' regulations and syllabus. The answers have been placed opposite the questions to stop the eternal page turning that exists with conventional texts. We think that this will make it easier to self-test. The answers are presented, we feel, in a helpful and constructive fashion.

We hope that the five examination papers in this book will help candidates to pass their final examination hurdle.

M. Brunner
P. N. Robinson
H. Williams

Introduction

The MCQ examination tests factual knowledge. It also tests breadth of knowledge, and therefore ensures that the whole syllabus is tested during the examination. The successful candidate will know the syllabus, which is freely available from the Royal College of Anaesthetists. It seems prudent to know what is required by the examiners!

These questions have been carefully constructed and the appropriate topics mixed to give a balanced subject range that will test, extend, and educate the reader. We have organized the text and answers to stop the candidate having to turn over several pages to find the answers. This will surely allow for better candidate attention and concentration when attempting these questions.

The scoring system is well known to everyone and this, of course, leads to the old chestnut questions. 'Should I guess if I haven't answered enough?' 'How many questions should be answered?' 'How many do I have to answer correctly to pass?' These questions are often asked. These are, as expected, impossible to answer to a candidate's satisfaction. We say outright guessing is not sensible and can lead to failure but that answers deduced from knowledge can often turn out to be correct. Answer as many questions as you can! There is no minimum number of answers acceptable and the examination is competitive. You have to aim to pass the multiple choice questions – a 1+ leaves no room for an error in any other part of the examination. It is best to consider that you are the potential 'gold medal' winner. Some candidates are always trying to 'get just enough marks to make it' and this is not a recommended attitude or an appropriate frame of mind. Suffice to say that it is best to get as many correct answers as you possibly can and to do that means a universal concise knowledge of anaesthesia.

The questions are of varying length. Some have stems of one word whilst others have complicated statements relating to the topic. The simple stems generally test a simple fact, such as a side effect of a drug. The complicated stems assess an ability to deduce facts from basic core knowledge. Some, as in the exam, are easy to read and some appear very complex. Read the questions and stems carefully!

The whole syllabus is covered in this text and knowledge and technique will, we hope, improve as a result of doing these multiple choice questions. We have constructed 5 balanced examination papers. This consists of 450 questions. We trust that the reader will indulge us in reading the 451st question!

Paper 1

1. The larynx
   A. Blood supply to the larynx is derived from the internal carotid artery
   B. The posterior cricoarytenoid muscle adducts the vocal cords
   C. The recurrent laryngeal nerve supplies all intrinsic muscles of the larynx
   D. The sternothyroid muscle depresses the larynx
   E. Thyrohyoid is supplied by the recurrent laryngeal nerve

2. Adenosine
   A. Increases oxygen consumption
   B. Increases coronary blood flow
   C. Slows atrioventricular conduction by increasing cellular permeability to calcium and reducing cellular permeability to potassium
   D. Has a half-life of 20 s
   E. May cause bronchospasm

3. Brainstem death
   A. Mydriasis is a feature
   B. Is associated with hypothermia
   C. Leads to asystole
   D. An oscillating pattern on transcranial Doppler is diagnostic
   E. Diabetes insipidus ensues

4. The following are recognized complications of the lithotomy position
   A. Saphenous nerve injury
   B. Peroneal nerve injury
   C. Obturator nerve injury
   D. Femoral nerve injury
   E. Lower limb compartment syndrome

1. **FFFTF**
   The blood supply to the larynx is derived from the superior and inferior thyroid arteries which are branches of the external carotid artery and thyrocervical trunk respectively. The posterior cricoarytenoid muscle is the only muscle to abduct the cords. The recurrent laryngeal nerve supplies all intrinsic muscles except the cricothyroid muscle. Sternothyroid depresses the larynx. Thyrohyoid is supplied by fibres from C1 conveyed in the hypoglossal nerve.

2. **FTFTT**
   Adenosine reduces oxygen consumption, increases coronary blood flow and slows atrioventricular conduction by reducing calcium and increasing potassium conductance. It is used to treat SVT and is less negatively inotropic than verapamil. Initially 3 mg IV is given, followed by 6 mg and 12 mg if necessary. Side effects include flushing and nausea, and bronchoconstriction in asthmatics.

3. **FTTTT**
   Mydriasis is not a feature of brainstem death; the pupils are usually in the mid-position. The body temperature falls after brain death due to vasodilatation, reduced metabolic rate and reduced muscle contraction. Brain death invariably leads to asystole. Although not a part of the UK criteria for diagnosis, an oscillating pattern on transcranial Doppler shows intracranial circulatory arrest and hence brainstem death. Resultant deficiency of ADH leads to diabetes insipidus.

4. **TTTTT**
   In the lithotomy position the saphenous nerve may be injured by compression against the medial tibial condyle. The common peroneal nerve may be injured by compression against the head of the fibula. The obturator nerve may be injured by excessive flexion at the hip joint. Injury to the femoral nerve may arise from hip flexion such that the inguinal ligament is stretched, thus compressing the nerve.

5. One atmosphere of pressure is equal to
A. $101\,325\,N/m^2$
B. $1033\,cm\,H_2O$
C. 760 Torr
D. $101\,325\,dyne/cm^2$
E. $14.7\,lb/in^2$

6. Features suggestive of smoke inhalation include
A. Heat injury to lung parenchyma
B. Burns within the oral cavity
C. Hoarse voice
D. Stridor
E. Sloughing off of pharyngeal mucosa

7. The following statements are true of the muscular dystrophies
A. Dystrophica myotonica is an X-linked recessive disease
B. Duchenne muscular dystrophy starts in childhood
C. Dystrophica myotonica patients can die suddenly due to cardiac conduction defects
D. Familial periodic paralysis syndromes are associated with abnormalities of potassium
E. Cataracts occur in patients with dystrophica myotonica

8. PEEP
A. Reduces myocardial wall tension
B. Lowers total lung water
C. Increases total lung capacity
D. An increased mixed venous oxygen tension indicates effectiveness
E. May increase dead space

5. **TTTFT**
The dyne is the force required to accelerate 1 g at a rate of 1 cm per second per second and is equal to 10^{-5} N. Following on: $1\,N/m^2 = 10^5\,dyne/10^4\,cm^2 = 10\,dyne/cm^2$. Unlike the millimetre of mercury, the Torr is independent of such variables as the density of mercury at different temperatures and pressures.

6. **FTTTT**
Heat injury to the lung parenchyma is not a feature because of the low specific heat capacity of smoke. The remaining features are suggestive of smoke inhalation.

7. **FTTTT**
Dystrophica myotonia has autosomal dominant inheritance and includes distal muscle wasting, frontal balding, cataracts, ptosis and myocardial conduction defects, which can be a cause of sudden death.

8. **TFFTT**
PEEP lowers the transmural pressure across the ventricle which, in accordance with Laplace's law, decreases myocardial wall tension. PEEP is effective in redistributing total lung water rather than lowering the amount present. PEEP increases FRC. An increased mixed venous oxygen tension is a good indicator of the effectiveness of PEEP. High levels of PEEP may increase dead space.

9. The following gases or vapours are attracted into a magnetic field (paramagnetic)
   A. Halothane
   B. Nitrogen
   C. Carbon dioxide
   D. Oxygen
   E. Nitric oxide

10. Nutritional requirements in adults
   A. Protein requirements are 1.5–2.0 g/kg/day
   B. Nitrogen requirements are 0.2 g/kg/day
   C. Phosphate requirements are 1.0–1.5 mmol/kg/day
   D. Magnesium requirements are 0.1–0.2 mmol/kg/day
   E. Glucose requirements are 4–5 g/kg/day

11. Regarding phosphate metabolism
   A. Phosphate is the dominant intracellular anion
   B. Normal plasma phosphate concentration is 0.8–1.5 mmol/l
   C. Hypophosphataemia is a complication of parenteral nutrition
   D. Hyperphosphataemia is associated with ectopic calcium deposition
   E. Acidosis causes hypophosphataemia

12. The following statements regarding the brachial plexus are true
   A. The brachial plexus is formed from the anterior primary rami of C5–T1
   B. The divisions of the brachial plexus lie within the interscalene groove
   C. The radial nerve lies inferior to the axillary artery in the axilla
   D. The musculocutaneous nerve arises from the terminal branch of the medial cord
   E. The terminal branch of the lateral cord forms the ulnar nerve

9. FFFTT
All gases are affected by magnetic fields. However, only two, oxygen and nitric oxide, are strongly paramagnetic. The other gases are weakly diamagnetic (i.e. repelled by a magnetic field). Paramagnetic oxygen gas analysers use the paramagnetic properties of oxygen.

10. FTFTT
Protein requirements are 0.5–1.0 g/kg/day.
Nitrogen: 0.2 g/kg/day.
Phosphate: 0.2–0.5 mmol/kg/day.
Magnesium: 0.1–0.2 mmol/kg/day.
Glucose: 4–5 g/kg/day.

11. TTTTF
The causes of hypophosphataemia are the same as those of hypokalaemia, i.e. alkalosis, insulin, β_2 agonists and glucose. Extracellular phosphate is redistributed intracellularly. It is therefore a complication of parenteral nutrition with a high carbohydrate content, especially when insulin is being administered. Other causes of hypophosphataemia are hyperparathyroidism and hypomagnesaemia. As the kidney maintains phosphate homeostasis, hypophosphataemia occurs if renal loss is excessive, whereas hyperphosphataemia is caused by renal failure. If the concentration of phosphate (mmol/l) multiplied by the concentration of calcium (mmol/l) is greater than six, ectopic calcification occurs.

12. TFFFF
The roots and trunks lie within the interscalene groove. In the axilla the radial nerve lies posterior to the axillary artery. The terminal branch of the lateral cord forms the musculocutaneous nerve. The terminal branch of the medial cord forms the ulnar nerve.

13. The porphyrias
  A. Acute intermittent porphyria is due to a defect with the mitochondrial enzyme porphobilinogen deaminase
  B. Acute intermittent porphyria exhibits photosensitivity
  C. Porphyria cutanea tarda may be acquired
  D. Acute intermittent porphyria has an equal sex distribution
  E. Hepatic porphyrias usually present in childhood

14. Concerning the glass pH electrode
  A. The reference electrode contains a calomel electrode connected to the test solution via a salt bridge (3.5 M KCl) solution
  B. The glass electrode develops a potential which is proportional to the hydrogen ion concentration in the test solution
  C. The reference electrode maintains a constant potential which varies only with temperature
  D. At 37°C, the glass electrode produces approximately 60 mV potential per pH unit change
  E. The pH electrode is connected to a pH meter which consists of a Wheatstone bridge circuit

15. Aldosterone secretion is significantly increased by
  A. ACTH
  B. Prostaglandin E
  C. Bradykinin
  D. Angiotensin II
  E. Hyponatraemia

13. FFTFF
Acute intermittent porphyria (AIP) is due to a defect in porphobilinogen deaminase, which is a cytosolic enzyme. AIP results in increased formation of delta aminolaevulinic acid and porphobilinogen. Cutaneous photosensitivity is a result of accumulation of preformed porphyrins. In AIP, porphyrin precursors accumulate and consequently photosensitivity is not a feature. Porphyria cutanea tarda may be familial or may arise in individuals exposed to polyhalogenated hydrocarbons. AIP is more common in females. The hepatic porphyrias rarely present before puberty.

14. TTTTF
The pH meter does not form part of a Wheatstone bridge circuit. The change in voltage relates to the pH of the test solution.

15. FTFTT
The main stimulus to aldosterone production is the renin–angiotensin mechanism via angiotensin II. Corticotrophin (ACTH) causes a small, but clinically insignificant, increase in aldosterone. People deficient in ACTH will have a low plasma cortisol level but a normal aldosterone level. Hyperkalaemia increases aldosterone secretion in addition to the factors mentioned in the question by a direct effect of potassium ions on the adrenocortical cells.

16. **Regarding diabetes mellitus, which of the following statements are correct**
    A. Maturity-onset diabetes of the young (MODY) presents before 25 years of age and is inherited as an autosomal recessive condition
    B. Fibrocalculous pancreatic diabetes mellitus (FPDM) is associated with obesity
    C. Chlorthalidone is a cause of secondary diabetes mellitus
    D. Mechanisms that lead to the development of neuropathy include myoinositol depletion
    E. The oral glucose tolerance test consists of the oral administration of a fixed dose of carbohydrate, this dose being generally agreed as 7.5 g

17. **Inhaled nitric oxide**
    A. Lowers peripheral vascular resistance
    B. Increases blood flow to both ventilated and non-ventilated areas of lung
    C. Mediates vasodilatation by increasing intracellular concentrations of cAMP
    D. Tachyphylaxis occurs after 1 week of therapy
    E. Nitrogen dioxide has bronchodilator properties

18. **Regarding peripheral neuropathy the following are correct**
    A. The commonest cause worldwide is leprosy
    B. It can be caused by rheumatoid arthritis
    C. Guillain–Barré syndrome typically begins with a distal paraesthesia and then progresses to motor syndromes
    D. Excesses of vitamins B1, B6, B12 and E are all causes of generalized peripheral neuropathy
    E. Nerve conduction velocity and EMG assessment distinguish the disease from primary muscle disease

16. FFTTF
MODY is inherited as an autosomal dominant condition and FPDM is associated with malnutrition. Chlorthalidone is a thiazide-related drug and hence can cause diabetes mellitus (as do steroids). Other mechanisms involved in the development of neuropathy include vascular abnormalities of the vasa nervorum and the accumulation of sorbitol. In diagnosing diabetes mellitus it is agreed that the dose should be 75 g. Glycosuria is suggestive, but not diagnostic, of diabetes mellitus and the diagnosis can be confirmed by a random whole blood glucose concentration of >10.0 mmol/l.

17. FFFFF
Due to its rapid reaction with haemoglobin, inhaled nitric oxide is deactivated within the pulmonary circulation. Inhaled nitric oxide only increases blood flow to ventilated areas of lung. Vasodilatation is mediated by increasing intracellular cGMP levels. Tachyphylaxis is not a feature. Nitrogen dioxide is toxic, causing bronchoconstriction.

18. TTTFT
Vitamin deficiency states are associated with peripheral neuropathy. Other causes are classified into metabolic (diabetes, chronic renal failure, porphyria, amyloidosis), toxins (alcohol, lead, drugs), inflammatory, autoimmune, infective, hereditary and the non-metastatic complications of malignancy. Motor and sensory weakness (glove and stocking) occurs and often accompanies an autonomic failure.

19. **Concerning phaeochromocytoma**
    A. Treatment of hypotension occurring after ligation of the venous drainage of the tumour during surgery usually requires the use of an α-receptor agonist, e.g. phenylephrine
    B. A vanillyl mandelic acid level greater than three times that of normal is diagnostic of phaeochromocytoma
    C. Hypercalcaemia is associated with phaeochromocytoma
    D. Phaeochromocytoma is associated with hyperglycaemia because catecholamines cause α_1-receptor-mediated inhibition of insulin release
    E. Somatostatin inhibits the release of catecholamines from phaeochromocytoma

20. **The following statements concerning the wavelengths of electromagnetic radiation are correct**
    A. Metres and greater = radio waves
    B. 680–6000 nm = infrared radiation
    C. 0.01–10 nm = ultraviolet radiation
    D. 10–680 nm = visible light
    E. mm–metres = diathermy

21. **Isoprenaline**
    A. Stimulates β and α_2 receptors
    B. Has no effect on the pulmonary vasculature
    C. Causes peripheral vasodilatation
    D. Increases myocardial oxygen demand
    E. Arrhythmias are uncommon

22. **Following aspiration of salt water in cases of near drowning**
    A. Lung compliance decreases
    B. Haemolysis occurs due to osmotic shifts
    C. Hypernatraemia often develops
    D. Cerebral oedema can occur
    E. Bicarbonate therapy is useful

19. FTTFT

Hypotension following ligation of the venous drainage of the tumour usually responds to fluid therapy guided by invasive pressure monitoring. A vanillyl mandelic acid level greater than three times normal is usually diagnostic of phaeochromocytoma. Hypercalcaemia is due either to associated parathyroid hyperplasia as part of multiple endocrine neoplasia, or to the secretion of a substance by the phaeochromocytoma, which promotes bone reabsorption. Raised plasma catecholamine levels cause an α_2-mediated inhibition of insulin release and antagonism of its action.

20. TTFFT

It is important to know these values as they are easy to ask in MCQs and often crop up in questions about monitoring, e.g. oximetry. As well as the values in the question, the following are also correct: $0.01–10\,nm$ = X-rays, $10–380\,nm$ = ultraviolet, $380–680\,nm$ = visible light.

21. FFTTF

Isoprenaline is purely a β agonist. It causes pulmonary and peripheral vasodilatation and increases heart rate and cardiac output. Arrhythmias are common.

22. TFFTT

Aspiration of seawater causes a reduction in lung compliance. Significant haemolysis is seen experimentally after aspiration of large quantities of fresh water but is not seen clinically. Hypernatraemia is not a feature of either. Resultant hypoxaemia can cause cerebral oedema. Lactic acidosis may require bicarbonate therapy.

23. Glycine as used for transurethral resection
  A. Is an essential amino acid
  B. Is reduced to form ammonia
  C. Absorption from the venous sinuses occurs at a rate of 10–30 ml/min
  D. Toxic effects occur as a consequence of ammonia formation
  E. Is used as a 2.2% solution

24. Concerning the pituitary gland
  A. Most pituitary tumours are hormone-secreting tumours which usually secrete growth hormone
  B. Patients with a growth hormone-secreting tumour often have an associated goitre
  C. Following operative pituitary surgery, diabetes insipidus is suggested if the patient has a plasma osmolality >295 mosmol/kg and a urine osmolality of >600 mosmol/kg
  D. Prolactin excess is associated with abnormal liver function tests in 25% of patients
  E. Hypopituitarism is associated with hypoglycaemia, an increased sensitivity to sedatives, pericardial effusion and low-voltage ECG changes

25. Regarding compliance
  A. Total thoracic compliance is equal to the sum of chest wall compliance and lung compliance
  B. Normal lung compliance is 1.5–2 l/kPa (150–200 ml/cmH_2O)
  C. Total thoracic compliance is 2.5–3 l/kPa (250–300 ml/cmH_2O)
  D. At normal tidal volumes the pressure/volume curve for lung compliance is approximately linear
  E. At lung volumes close to the functional residual capacity (FRC) the change in lung volume for a given change in pressure is greater during inflation of the lungs than during deflation

23. FFTTF
Glycine is a non-essential amino acid. It is oxidatively deaminated in the liver, producing ammonia. Absorption rates are estimated to be 10–30 ml/min. Toxic effects occur directly due to glycine (visual defects) and as a result of its conversion to ammonia (malaise, nausea and vomiting). Glycine is presented for this use as a 1.5% solution.

24. FTFFT
Most pituitary tumours are non-secreting. Of the hormone-secreting tumours the majority secrete growth hormone or prolactin. The goitre that occurs with acromegaly results from direct stimulation of the thyroid gland by growth hormone and is non-toxic. Diabetes insipidus is suggested if the plasma osmolality is >295 mosmol/kg and the urine osmolality is <300 mosmol/kg. Prolactin excess is not associated with any medical or anaesthetic considerations. Hypopituitarism is also associated with hypothyroidism, which can cause hypoglycaemia, hypoadrenalism and other ECG changes, such as prolonged PR and QT intervals.

25. FTFTF
1/total thoracic compliance = 1/chest wall compliance + 1/lung compliance.
Total thoracic compliance = 0.85 l/kPa (85 ml/cmH$_2$O). The volume change of the lung for a given change in pressure is greater during deflation than inflation, resulting in the hysteresis seen on pressure/volume curves. Hysteresis is due to the effects of surface tension.

26. Concerning tetanus
   A. *Clostridium tetani* is a Gram-negative organism
   B. Tetanus exotoxin migrates along motor nerves to the posterior horn cells in the spinal cord
   C. Labetalol is a useful treatment
   D. Isolated trismus requires the passage of a nasogastric tube to prevent aspiration
   E. The incubation period is usually <15 days

27. Horner's syndrome
   A. Results from interruption of the sympathetic fibres en route from the eye
   B. Has miosis and exophthalmos as components
   C. Has ptosis as a feature because there is loss of the sympathetic pseudomotor fibres
   D. Has contralateral loss of facial sweating
   E. Can accompany brainstem infarct

28. Concerning the use of Hartmann's solution
   A. Hartmann's solution contains 131 mmol/l sodium ions
   B. Hartmann's solution contains 19 mmol/l lactate ions
   C. Metabolism of lactate yields predominantly bicarbonate ions
   D. Oxidation of lactate yields glucose
   E. Metabolism of lactate yields hydrogen ions

29. Cimetidine interacts with the following drugs
   A. Warfarin
   B. Theophylline
   C. Phenytoin
   D. Amiodarone
   E. Metformin

26. FFTFT

C. tetani is a Gram-positive organism. Tetanus exotoxin migrates along motor nerves to the anterior horn cells in the spinal cord. Labetalol has been successfully used in cases of sympathetic overactivity, which is often a feature. In cases of isolated trismus, nasogastric tubes should be avoided as stimulation can cause laryngospasm. In 90% of cases the incubation period is <15 days.

27. FFFFT

Horner's syndrome results from interruption of the sympathetic fibres to the pupil. A feature is enophthalmus. The ptosis is due to paralysis of Muller's muscle. Ipsilateral loss of facial sweating occurs. The miosis is best detected in a dark room to emphasize the pupillary difference. The causes include brainstem infarction and haemorrhage, outflow at T1 blockade as in stellate ganglion block, brachial plexus and Pancoast tumour, and lesions of the carotid artery such as dissection.

28. TFFFF

Hartmann's solution contains 131 mmol/l sodium ions and 29 mmol/l lactate ions. The metabolism of lactate is mostly hepatic. Seventy per cent is converted to glucose by gluconeogenesis and 30% is converted to bicarbonate by oxidation. Both reactions utilize hydrogen ions.

29. TTTFT

Cimetidine binds to cytochrome P_{450}, causing enzymatic inhibition and prolonging the effects of warfarin, phenytoin and theophyllines. Cimetidine impairs the excretion of metformin.

30. The intra-aortic balloon pump
   A. Inflates during systole
   B. Raises aortic diastolic pressure
   C. Is triggered by the patient's ECG
   D. Is partially effective in the absence of a beating heart
   E. May precipitate aortic dissection

31. Subarachnoid haemorrhage
   A. Is more common in people >65 years of age
   B. The diagnosis is confirmed if appropriate CT scanning is performed after 2 days
   C. CT scanning will pick up all aneurysms
   D. Antifibrinolytic drugs are the mainstay of therapy
   E. Calcium channel entry blockers cause vasospasm

32. Endotoxin
   A. The A antigen is responsible for the biological activity
   B. Is responsible for toxic shock syndrome
   C. Is only found in Gram-negative organisms
   D. Monoclonal antibodies have been raised against the O antigens
   E. Stimulates the alternative complement pathway

33. Concerning insulin
   A. Insulin is required by brain, liver and muscle for the uptake of glucose
   B. Insulin decreases circulating levels of fatty acids, glycerol and amino acids
   C. Isophane insulin consists of insulin complexed with protamine to prolong its duration of action
   D. In humans, 120 g of glucose can be absorbed from the intestine per hour
   E. Only the liver contains glucose-6-phosphatase and it is therefore the only organ capable of storing glucose as glycogen

30. **FTTFT**
The intra-aortic balloon pump inflates during diastole raising aortic diastolic pressure. The inflation–deflation sequence is initiated by the patient's ECG. As an assist device it is useless in the absence of a beating heart. A recognized complication is acute aortic dissection.

31. **TFFFF**
SAH accounts for 5% of all strokes. Appropriate CT scanning confirms the diagnosis if performed within 48 h of the onset of symptoms. CT scanning misses small aneurysms. Antifibrinolytic drugs are never used in the treatment of subarachnoid haemorrhage because, although they reduce the risk of re-bleeding, they increase the risk of cerebral infarction. Calcium blockers are used to prevent vasospasm.

32. **TFTFT**
The A antigen is responsible for the biological activity of endotoxin. Exotoxins produced by *Staphylococcus aureus* are responsible for the toxic shock syndrome. Endotoxin is only produced by Gram-negative organisms. Because of structural conservation between species, monoclonal antibodies have been raised against the A antigen. Endotoxin stimulates the alternative complement pathway.

33. **FTFTF**
The brain, unlike muscle and liver, does not require insulin for the uptake of glucose. The liver is the only organ which contains glucose-6-phosphatase. It is the only organ, therefore, which can liberate glucose from glycogen into the circulation. Other organs, e.g. muscle, can also store glycogen but are only able to utilize it locally.

34. Acid-base management during hypothermic cardiopulmonary bypass
  A. Hypothermia lowers blood pH
  B. Alpha-stat management of blood gases requires the administration of exogenous carbon dioxide to the oxygenator
  C. The cerebral circulatory response to carbon dioxide tension is preserved during hypothermia
  D. pH-stat management increases cerebral blood flow
  E. Alpha-stat management requires temperature correction of blood gases

35. Concerning local anaesthetic nerve blocks of the leg
  A. The sciatic nerve is derived from the L4–S3 nerve roots of the sacral plexus
  B. The femoral nerve is purely sensory and supplies skin over the medial lower leg and foot via the saphenous branch
  C. The lateral cutaneous nerve of the thigh is a branch of the femoral nerve
  D. The 'three-in-one block' anaesthetizes the femoral, sciatic and obturator nerves
  E. The genitofemoral nerve is formed from the anterior primary rami of L1–L2

36. The following treatments are of use in amitriptyline poisoning
  A. IV isoprenaline
  B. IV disopyramide
  C. IV digoxin
  D. IV sodium bicarbonate
  E. Haemofiltration

34. FFTTF
Hypothermia causes a rise in the blood pH due to the increased solubility (and hence decreased partial pressure) of carbon dioxide. pH-stat management of blood gases aims to keep pH at 7.4 at the patient's core temperature which requires the administration of exogenous carbon dioxide to the oxygenator. As the cerebral circulatory response to carbon dioxide tension is maintained during hypothermia, pH-stat management leads to an increased cerebral blood flow. Alpha-stat management maintains a non-temperature-corrected pH of 7.4 and a PCO_2 of 5.3 kPa.

35. TFFFT
The femoral nerve supplies muscles of the hip and knee as well as the skin over the medial lower leg and foot via the saphenous branch. The lateral cutaneous nerve of the thigh arises directly from the lumbar plexus (L2–L3). The 'three-in-one block' anaesthetizes the femoral, lateral cutaneous and obturator nerves, providing analgesia to the anterior thigh.

36. TFFTF
Amitriptyline in overdose has a quinidine (class 1A)-like effect on the heart, prolonging the QT interval and potentially causing torsade de pointes. Isoprenaline may be useful as it shortens the QT interval. The administration of other class 1A drugs should be avoided. Digoxin should also be avoided as it increases a tendency to heart block. A priority in the treatment of arrhythmias caused by amitriptyline overdose is aggressive treatment of acidosis with sodium bicarbonate. Haemofiltration is not useful, as amitriptyline is highly lipid-soluble and 95–99% protein-bound.

37. In multiple sclerosis
  A.   Loss of function in part of the nervous system is associated with a rise in body temperature
  B.   Dantrolene can be used for spasticity
  C.   Onset normally occurs between 20 and 40 years of age and the disease occurs more commonly in the tropical regions of the world
  D.   The myelin sheath of neurones in the peripheral nerves is affected
  E.   A serum vitamin B12 test needs to be performed to exclude subacute combined degeneration of the spinal cord as part of the differential diagnosis of the disease

38. Suxamethonium
  A.   May be administered safely in amyotrophic lateral sclerosis
  B.   Onset time is increased in the presence of atypical cholinesterase
  C.   Onset time is more rapid in adductor pollicus than in the laryngeal adductors
  D.   Is potentiated by aminophylline
  E.   Lowers intragastric pressure

39. Concerning leukotrienes
  A.   Leukotrienes are formed from prostaglandins in response to various immunological stimuli
  B.   Leukotrienes are released from mast cells, leucocytes and erythrocytes
  C.   Ketanserin inhibits the synthesis of the leukotriene LTC_4, which is a mediator of anaphylaxis
  D.   The leukotriene LTB_4 is a potent chemotactic agent for other cells involved in the inflammatory response
  E.   Non-steroidal anti-inflammatory drugs (NSAIDs) inhibit the synthesis of all leukotrienes

37. **TTFFT**
The disease affects the myelin sheath of neurones in the CNS, not those of peripheral nerves. The disease occurs more commonly in temperate climates and about 70% of patients are female. The disease commonly affects the periventricular deep white matter, the optic nerve, the brainstem and the spinal cord.

38. **FTFTF**
Amyotrophic lateral sclerosis is a form of neurogenic muscle atrophy disease of the corticospinal tracts. Use of suxamethonium may result in severe hyperkalaemia. Suxamethonium onset has been shown to be slower in the presence of atypical variants of plasma cholinesterase. The onset of action of suxamethonium is more rapid at the larnygeal adductors than the adductor pollicus. Suxamethonium raises intragastric pressure.

39. **FFFTF**
Leukotrienes are formed from the effect of lipoxygenase on arachidonic acid in response to thermal, chemical and infective, as well as immunological, stimuli. Leukotrienes are released from leucocytes, platelets and mast cells. Ketanserin is a 5-HT$_2$ and α-receptor antagonist. NSAIDs block the effect of cyclo-oxygenase on arachidonic acid, which is responsible for the synthesis of prostaglandins, prostacyclin and thromboxanes.

40. 'A' waves during the measurement of intracranial pressure
   A.   Are associated with an intracranial pressure >10 mmHg
   B.   Indicate that spatial compensation is exhausted
   C.   Have a maximum amplitude of 100 mmHg
   D.   Have a duration of 2–5 min
   E.   Are not of prognostic significance

41. In tetralogy of Fallot there is
   A.   A ventriculoseptal defect
   B.   An aorta overriding the defect which receives blood
         from both the right and left ventricles
   C.   Pulmonary stenosis
   D.   Right ventricular hypertrophy
   E.   Squatting in children decreases the right-to-left shunt of
         blood through the ventriculoseptal defect

42. Trigeminal neuralgia
   A.   Affects men and women with equal frequency
   B.   The maxillary division is affected most commonly
   C.   Allodynia is rarely a feature
   D.   Is often caused by underlying organic pathology
   E.   May be treated by glycerol injection into the trigeminal
         ganglion

40. FTTFF
'A' waves are associated with an intracranial pressure >20 mmHg. Their presence indicates that spatial compensation is exhausted. They have a maximum amplitude of 100 mmHg and a duration of 10–15 min. They are of prognostic significance.

41. TTTTT
Management is directed towards medical and surgical remedies. Acute hypoxic crises with severe cyanosis can be treated with noradrenaline to increase systemic vascular resistance, and morphine or propranolol to relax the infundibulum. Total surgical correction is possible but depends upon the size of the pulmonary artery. Failing total correction, systemic to pulmonary artery shunts are used. Squatting in children kinks the femoral arteries, increases the systemic vascular resistance and decreases the right-to-left shunt of blood through the ventriculoseptal defect.

42. FFFFT
Trigeminal neuralgia affects females almost twice as commonly as males. The mandibular division is most frequently involved. Allodynia is a frequent feature. An underlying organic cause, such as tumour or multiple sclerosis, occurs in only 1–5% of cases. When drug therapy is ineffective glycerol can be injected into the trigeminal ganglion.

43. **In patients with pre-eclampsia**
    A. Platelet concentration is reduced due to increased levels of plasma thromboxane
    B. Prothrombin time and platelet count are the most reliable tests of clotting
    C. In order to prevent convulsions, therapeutic blood levels of magnesium should be 1–2 mmol/l
    D. Fibrinogen concentration falls significantly due to increased consumption
    E. Magnesium overdose causes ECG changes and loss of deep tendon reflexes when the plasma concentration exceeds 7 mmol/l

44. **Concerning azeotropes**
    A. An azeotrope is a mixture of liquids which forms a precipitate when mixed in specific ratios by volume
    B. Azeotropes cannot be separated by distillation
    C. Halothane and ether form an azeotrope when mixed in a ratio of 2:1
    D. Propofol is an example of an azeotrope
    E. The boiling point of each liquid forming an azeotrope is altered by the presence of the others

45. **The following are associated with convulsions in overdose or poisoning**
    A. Isoniazid
    B. Cyanide
    C. Carbon monoxide
    D. Digoxin
    E. Glibenclamide

46. **Regarding atrial fibrillation**
    A. No apparent cause is found in 40% of patients
    B. It can be caused by re-entry bypass tracts such as in the Wolff–Parkinson–White (WPW) syndrome
    C. It can be caused by hypothyroidism
    D. It can be caused by acute alcohol intoxication
    E. It can be caused by post-operative pneumonia

43. TFFFF
Plasma fibrinogen concentration is unaltered unless there is a concomitant placental abruption when it is greatly reduced. Bleeding time is the most reliable test of clotting in pre-eclampsia. Therapeutic blood levels of magnesium are 2–3 mmol/l. These are achieved by administering a bolus dose of 4 g of magnesium sulphate over 5 min, followed by an infusion of 1–2 g/h. ECG abnormalities occur when the plasma concentration is >2.5 mmol/l, deep tendon reflexes are lost at levels >5 mmol/l, respiratory arrest occurs at 7 mmol/l and cardiac arrest at 12–15 mmol/l. Magnesium is a popular topic and needs to be known in depth!

44. FTTFT
An azeotrope is a mixture of liquids whose components cannot be separated by distillation. The boiling point of each liquid in an azeotropic mixture is changed so that their boiling points become identical. A eutectic mixture is a mixture in which the melting point of each component is lowered. In the case of a eutectic mixture of lignocaine and prilocaine (EMLA) the resulting substance forms a solid.

45. TTTFT
In overdose isoniazid decreases GABA synthesis leading to CNS stimulation. Both cyanide and carbon monoxide cause fitting by hypoxic mechanisms. The hypoglycaemia associated with glibenclamide overdose is a cause of fitting.

46. TTFTT
It can be caused by hyperthyroidism. The discharge of the atrium can be as high as 500 beats per minute. The WPW syndrome is due to a congenital accessory bundle, the Bundle of Kent, which is between the atrium and the ventricular myocardium. The ventricular myocardium depolarizes early, leading to early deflection in the QRS complex and this is the delta wave.

47. Remifentanil
   A. Is partially antagonized by naloxone
   B. $t_{1/2elim}$ is 3–5 min
   C. Is 70% protein-bound
   D. Has a volume of distribution higher than that of alfentanil
   E. Is metabolized by red cell esterases

48. Regarding carbon dioxide
   A. Carbon dioxide is supplied in grey cylinders with black shoulders
   B. Carbon dioxide has a critical temperature of $-31°C$
   C. At room temperature the pressure in a full carbon dioxide cylinder is 150 bar
   D. Carbon dioxide is less dense than air
   E. Carbon dioxide is manufactured by mixing magnesium carbonate with a strong acid

49. Dopexamine
   A. Should be administered only via a central vein
   B. Stimulates β_1 receptors directly
   C. Stimulates α receptors indirectly
   D. Has beneficial effects on splanchnic perfusion
   E. Increases pulmonary capillary wedge pressure

50. Regarding examination of the JVP
   A. In atrial fibrillation the 'a' wave is lost
   B. Cannon waves are huge 'a' waves which are due to atrial contraction against a closed tricuspid valve
   C. In cardiac tamponade only the 'x' descent is prominent
   D. The 'v' wave is due to right atrial filling against a closed tricuspid valve
   E. The 'c' wave may be visible immediately after the 'a' wave and is due to right ventricular contraction filling the right atrium before the tricuspid valve is closed

47. **FFTFT**
Remifentanil is fully antagonized by naloxone. It has a $t_{1/2elim}$ of 9.5 min. Remifentanil is 70% plasma protein-bound to α_1 acid glycoprotein. Due to the degree of protein binding it has a lower volume of distribution than other opioids. Remifentanil is metabolized by both tissue and red cell esterases.

48. **FFFFF**
Carbon dioxide is 1.5 times denser than air, has a molecular weight of 44, a boiling point of $-19°C$ and a critical temperature of $+31°C$. It is manufactured by heating calcium or magnesium carbonate and is supplied in grey cylinders with grey shoulders. The pressure in a full carbon dioxide cylinder at room temperature is 57 bar.

49. **FFFTF**
Dopexamine is administered as an infusion via a central vein or a large peripheral vein. It is a potent agonist at β_2 receptors and an indirect stimulator of β_1 receptors. It has no significant activity at α receptors. Dopexamine has beneficial effects on the splanchnic circulation. Pulmonary capillary wedge pressure is lowered by dopexamine.

50. **TTTTT**
The clinical examination of venous pressure is important. There are three peaks and two descents in a normal venous pressure in every cardiac cycle. The main abnormalities are presented correctly in the question.

51. The following changes occur in the respiratory system in pregnancy at term
A.   Airway resistance increases
B.   Total lung capacity remains unchanged
C.   Vital capacity decreases
D.   Dead space increases
E.   Inspiratory capacity decreases

52. Cardioplegia solution used in cardiac surgery contains
A.   Greater than 140 mmol/l sodium ions
B.   Approximately 15 mmol/l potassium chloride to cause cardiac arrest in diastole on infusion into the coronary arteries
C.   Magnesium 5 mmol/l to prevent the entry of calcium into myocardial cells
D.   Prilocaine 0–1 mmol/l to reduce post-bypass arrhythmias
E.   Mannitol to prevent water accumulation during cardiac bypass

53. Clinical features that allow the diagnosis of systemic inflammatory response syndrome to be made include
A.   Systolic blood pressure <90 mmHg
B.   pH <7.15
C.   Temperature <36°C
D.   Underlying sepsis
E.   Bicarbonate <15 mmol/l

54. A sixth cranial nerve palsy
A.   Is caused by diabetes mellitus in the elderly
B.   Is most commonly caused by multiple sclerosis in the young
C.   Can be indicative of dysthyroid eye disease
D.   Results in failure to adduct the eye
E.   When it occurs bilaterally myasthenia gravis should be suspected

51. FFFFF
The airway resistance decreases due to dilatation of the airways below the larynx. Total lung capacity decreases by 5%. Vital capacity remains unchanged. Dead space is unaltered. The inspiratory capacity increases by 15%.

52. FTFFT
Cardioplegia solution contains:
110–140 mmol/l NaCl ions, to prevent water accumulation.
10–20 mmol/l KCl.
16 mmol/l $MgCl_2$ and 1.2–2.2 mmol/l $CaCl_2$ to protect against potassium damage post-bypass. The magnesium reduces calcium entry into myocardial cells.
0–1 mmol/l procaine reduces post-bypass arrhythmias.

53. FFTFF
Diagnosis of systemic inflammatory response syndrome can be made if two or more of the following features are present:
Temperature $>38°C$ or $<36°C$.
Heart rate >90 beats/min.
Respiratory rate >20 breaths/min or P_aCO_2 <4.3 kPa.
White blood cell count $>12\,000$ cells/mm^3 or <4000 cells/mm^3 or $>10\%$ immature band forms.

54. TTTFT
The nucleus of the sixth nerve lies in the floor of the fourth ventricle in direct contact with the CSF. It traverses the temporal bone before passing through the cavernous sinus to innervate the lateral rectus muscle of the eye. Palsy causes failure to abduct the eye. Diplopia is a common symptom. It can occur after lumbar puncture and is a rare complication of epidural dural puncture and spinal anaesthesia; however, the most common cause in the young is multiple sclerosis.

55. The following statements about α_2 agonists are true
  A. Dexmetetomidine lowers MAC by 50%
  B. Physiological effects are mediated by decreased intracellular cAMP
  C. Dexmetetomidine is inhibited by the pertussis toxin
  D. Clonidine has a $t_{1/2elim}$ of 2–3 h
  E. Intravenous α_2 agonists initially cause hypertension

56. When administering an anaesthetic using positive pressure ventilation and a closed circuit circle breathing system
  A. A Goldman vaporizer can be used
  B. A vaporizer outside the circle (VOC) can be used
  C. Dangerously high concentrations of anaesthetic vapour can be delivered to the patient
  D. At very low gas flow rates the concentration, within the breathing system, of anaesthetic vapours with higher blood solubility is less likely to increase than that of vapours with lower blood solubility
  E. Barium lime or soda lime must be used

57. Regarding the decontamination of anaesthetic equipment
  A. Chlorhexidine 0.1–0.5% is used as a disinfectant
  B. Gluteraldehyde 2% kills all organisms and spores
  C. Following the use of ethylene oxide, sterilized plastic anaesthetic apparatus should not be used for 2 days, in order to prevent toxic damage to the patient
  D. As the pressure within an autoclave is increased, the time required to sterilize equipment is reduced
  E. Pasteurization kills spores as well as bacteria

55. FFTFT
Dexmetetomidine lowers MAC by 90%. The physiological effects of α_2 agonists are mediated by an increase in intracellular cAMP. Clonidine has a $t_{1/2elim}$ of 9–12 h. Intravenous administration of α_2 agonists produces a biphasic response, initially stimulating post-junctional α_2 receptors in the peripheral vascular system and causing increased systemic vascular resistance and hypertension. This is followed by a longer-lasting drop in blood pressure mediated centrally.

56. TTTTT
The Goldman vaporizer is a draw-over vaporizer used inside the circle (VIC) during closed circuit anaesthesia. When the fresh gas flow rate is very low, e.g. 250 ml/min, the concentration of vapour within the circle system can rise to dangerously high levels. This is due to reduced anaesthetic uptake by the patient, which allows vapour to accumulate. The lower the blood solubility of the vapour, the less will be taken up by the patient, further increasing the concentration of the anaesthetic within the circuit. Accumulation of anaesthetic vapour is therefore less likely to occur with more soluble anaesthetics that are more abundantly taken up by the patient.

57. TFFTF
Disinfection, using substances such as 2% gluteraldehyde and 0.1–0.5% chlorhexidine and processes such as pasteurization, kills most organisms but not spores. Sterilization, using autoclave and ethylene oxide, kills all organisms and spores. Ethylene oxide is toxic and taken up by plastics. Equipment sterilized with ethylene oxide should not be used for 2 weeks.

58. Carbon monoxide poisoning
   A. Cherry red discolouration of mucous membranes is a common presenting feature
   B. May present with skin blistering
   C. Carbon monoxide has 100 times the affinity for haemoglobin than oxygen
   D. The half-life of carbon monoxide in room air is 4–6 h
   E. Gastrointestinal symptoms are a feature

59. Regarding asthma
   A. Asthma can be defined as reversible partial obstruction to airflow in the intrathoracic airways
   B. Bronchial hyperactivity of smooth muscle is seen in a small number of asthmatics
   C. Atopic individuals have increased levels of circulating IgE (the reaginic antibody) which binds to mast cells in the bronchial mucosa and lumen
   D. Eosinophilic major protein is not responsible for mucosal damage and shedding
   E. An improvement in FEV_1 or PEFR of at least 15–20% after inhaling a bronchodilator provides a diagnosis of asthma

60. Anaphylactic reactions and anaesthesia
   A. Thiopentone is the only anaesthetic agent associated with type IV hypersensitivity reactions
   B. The severity of anaphylactic shock is reduced in the beta-blocked patient
   C. Anaphylaxis is rare at extremes of age
   D. Plasma histamine levels of 15 nmol/l are suggestive of anaphylaxis
   E. Skin prick testing uses drugs diluted a thousand times

58. FTFTT
Cherry red discolouration is a rare feature indicating severe poisoning. Cyanosis and pallor are more usual. Skin blistering and bullae can occur as a result of hypoxia. The affinity of carbon monoxide for haemoglobin is 200–240 times that of oxygen. In room air the half-life of carbon monoxide by lung excretion is 4–6 h. Nausea, abdominal pain and diarrhoea are all features of carbon monoxide poisoning.

59. TFTFT
Bronchial hyper-reactivity is seen in nearly all asthmatics. Eosinophilic major basic protein is responsible for the mucosal damage. Asthma is important. When answering questions in vivas clear definitions are valuable. Asthma is one topic but other respiratory definitions that must be known include respiratory failure, adult respiratory distress syndrome, pneumothorax and chronic bronchitis. Asthma can be classified into allergenic or non-allergenic, and allergenic patients have high circulating levels of IgE. The management of asthma, especially status asthmaticus, occurs regularly in examination questions and candidates need to discuss the clinical signs, the best induction agent available, the place of magnesium, the types of ventilator available and the drug treatment commonly used.

60. TFTFF
The severity of anaphylactic reactions is increased in β-blocked patients. A plasma histamine level of 15 nmol/l is up to 100 times lower than the levels observed during anaphylaxis. Skin prick testing uses drugs in an undiluted form.

61. The following statements concerning gas analysis are true

   A.   The van Slyke apparatus depends on a reduction in overall pressure in a burette of the gas being measured as it reacts with other substances to produce a non-gaseous compound

   B.   The Dräger Narkotest depends on the absorption of ultraviolet light by halothane

   C.   The Hook and Tucker halothane meter depends on a change in tension of a rubber strip as halothane dissolves in it

   D.   Enflurane and isoflurane, but not halothane, absorb infrared light

   E.   The Dräger Narkotest is temperature compensated

62. The following are types of laryngoscope blade

   A.   Wisconsin
   B.   Seward
   C.   Soper
   D.   Brewer–Luckhardt
   E.   Bellhouse

63. Concerning ankylosing spondylitis

   A.   Chronic anaemia is not a feature
   B.   Aortic stenosis may occur and there are associated cardiac conduction defects
   C.   Bilateral upper lobe fibrosis may occur in the lungs
   D.   It occurs most commonly in Caucasian men aged between 15 and 40 years of age
   E.   Cauda equina syndrome is a late rare complication

61. **TFFFT**
To measure blood gases using the van Slyke apparatus, oxygen and carbon dioxide are liberated from blood into a burette, where they react with other substances to form non-gaseous substances. The fall in pressure of gas in the burette relates to the blood gases. The Haldane apparatus is similar to the van Slyke apparatus except that volume, rather than pressure change, is measured. The Hook and Tucker halothane meter depends on the ability of halothane to absorb ultraviolet light while the Dräger Narkotest, which is temperature-compensated, measures the reduction in tension of a rubber strip as halothane dissolves in it. Any gaseous substance made up of two or more different atoms, including all of the volatile agents as well as carbon dioxide and nitrous oxide, absorbs infrared light.

62. **TTTFT**
There are many different types of laryngoscope blade; those mentioned in the question are amongst the most common. The Bellhouse, for example, has an optical prism at the angle while the Wisconsin is similar to the Magill, with the bulb nearer the tip. One can look up pictures of these blades in anaesthetic textbooks. The Brewer–Luckhardt reflex is a reflex that results in laryngospasm following a distal stimulus, such as dilatation of the cervix.

63. **FFTTT**
Chronic anaemia is a feature. Aortic incompetence occurs with the disease and conduction defects also occur. The aetiology is unknown but a variety of organisms have been suggested, with *Klebsiella* a likely candidate. HLA-B27 seems to be a major susceptibility gene. Patients with this condition present with bone and joint features – lower back pain, asymmetrical peripheral arthritis and enthesitis (ligamentous bone junction arthritis resulting in pleuritic chest pain) – as well as systemic manifestations: eye, lungs and carditis.

64. Stellate ganglion block
   A. The stellate ganglion is formed from the seventh and eighth cervical sympathetic ganglia
   B. The stellate ganglion lies anterior to the carotid sheath
   C. Successful block is indicated by an ipsilateral mydriasis
   D. Successful block is indicated by ipsilateral nasal congestion
   E. Hoarse voice is a complication

65. Regarding medical gas cylinders
   A. The pressure in a full air cylinder is 13 700 kPa
   B. Helium is presented in brown cylinders with brown shoulders
   C. A full size E oxygen cylinder contains 680 l of oxygen
   D. Nitrous oxide, carbon dioxide and cyclopropane cylinders contain liquid at room temperature
   E. The pseudocritical temperature of entonox is dependent on the pressure in the cylinder

66. Concerning the ITU management of Guillain–Barré syndrome
   A. Plasma exchange has been shown to lower overall mortality
   B. Plasma exchange lowers the need for mechanical ventilation
   C. Bulbar involvement is an indication for intubation
   D. A vital capacity <30% of that predicted is an indication for intubation
   E. Sixty per cent of patients will require mechanical ventilation

64. **FFFTT**
The stellate ganglion is formed from the fusion of the
seventh and eighth cervical and the first thoracic sympathetic
ganglia. It lies posterior to the carotid sheath. Successful
stellate ganglion block is indicated by sympathetic
denervation of the head and neck. This causes both
ipsilateral nasal congestion and miosis. Local anaesthetic
solutions may spread to the ipsilateral recurrent laryngeal
nerve causing hoarseness.

65. **TTTTT**
Nitrous oxide, carbon dioxide and cyclopropane are vapours
at room temperature as they are below their critical
temperatures. Therefore, the cylinders will contain liquid and
vapour. The pseudocritical temperature is the temperature at
which a mixture of gases will separate into its component
parts. Pseudocritical temperature varies with pressure and is
$-7°C$ in entonox cylinders (135 bar) and $-30°C$ for pipelines
(4 bar).

66. **FTTTF**
Plasma exchange has been shown to reduce the likelihood of
patients requiring mechanical ventilation, but it does not
reduce overall mortality. Indications for intubation include
bulbar involvement and a vital capacity <30% of predicted.
In total, 20–30% of patients will require mechanical
ventilation.

67. Regarding the fetal circulation
  A. Systemic venous blood returns to the right atrium
  B. The pulmonary circulation is short circuited by both the patent ductus arteriosus and the foramen ovale
  C. On delivery the patent ductus arteriosus closes as a result of both lower levels of prostaglandins and oxygenated blood
  D. Adult haemoglobin begins to appear in the fetal circulation at 40 weeks' gestation and comprises 40% of the haemoglobin by the time of birth
  E. Mixed blood in the inferior vena cava has a saturation of 80%

68. The stress response to surgery results in
  A. Reduced protein synthesis
  B. A positive nitrogen balance
  C. Reduced levels of growth hormone
  D. Increased levels of vasopressin
  E. Reduced levels of T_3

69. The rate of diffusion of a gas across a membrane into a liquid
  A. Is proportional to the area of the membrane
  B. Is proportional to the square root of the molecular weight of the gas
  C. Decreases as the temperature of the liquid increases
  D. Is related to Graham's law
  E. Is inversely proportional to the density of the gas

67. TTTFF

Adult haemoglobin begins to appear in the fetal circulation at around 20 weeks' gestation and comprises 20% by the time of birth. This rises to 90% by the age of 4 months, as the body does not manufacture fetal haemoglobin after birth. Fetal blood leaving the placenta in the umbilical vein is 80% saturated – it mixes with systemic and portal blood and the resulting blood in the inferior vena cava has a saturation of about 67%. Fetal haemoglobin has gamma chains which replace the adult beta chains and bind 2,3-diphosphoglycerate less efficiently, leading to a greater affinity for oxygen than adult haemoglobin.

68. FFFTT

The liver responds to the stress response by increasing production of acute phase proteins, while production of albumin, retinol and transferrin is reduced. There is a negative nitrogen balance. Levels of growth hormone and vasopressin increase while levels of T_3 drop.

69. TFTTF

The rate of diffusion of a gas across a membrane into a liquid is proportional to the area of the membrane, the concentration gradient across the membrane and the solubility of the gas, and inversely proportional to the square root of the molecular weight of the gas (Graham's law). As the rate of diffusion is proportional to solubility, and solubility of a substance decreases as the temperature of the liquid in which it is dissolved increases, the rate of diffusion of a gas across a membrane into a liquid falls as the liquid increases in temperature.

70. **The following are appropriate in the management of fulminant hepatic failure**
    A. Prophylactic FFP
    B. Intracranial pressure monitoring
    C. IV dextrose 20%
    D. Early feeding with TPN
    E. Measurement of serum ceruloplasmin levels

71. **Cystic fibrosis**
    A. Has autosomal recessive inheritance
    B. Seventy per cent of cases are caused by the deltaF508 gene mutation on chromosome 7
    C. Sweat contains a high concentration of sodium which is due to an abnormality of chloride channel regulation at the cell luminal surface
    D. Recurrent *Staphylococcus aureus* infections are common and the respiratory tract is colonized by pseudomonas
    E. Diabetes mellitus is present in 90% of adults with the disease

72. **Clinical features of an intra-operative transfusion reaction include**
    A. Hypertension
    B. Fever
    C. Pruritus
    D. Increased bleeding at the operative site
    E. Dyspnoea

70. FTTFT

In the management of fulminant hepatic failure prophylactic FFP has not been shown to influence outcome favourably. Cerebral oedema associated with fulminant hepatic failure is optimally managed with intracranial pressure monitoring. Hypoglycaemia is a common feature, and is treated with infusions of 10% or 20% dextrose. This is all the nutritional therapy that should be given initially. Serum ceruloplasmin levels are diagnostic in Wilson's disease, a rare cause of fulminant hepatic failure.

71. TTTTF

With increasing age there is an increasing incidence of diabetes but it only presents in 20% of all adults. The abnormal chloride channel cell regulation also results in the low water content of mucus produced by airways, the pancreas and the intestine. Haematological investigations are usually normal but sweat sodium levels are elevated to >70 mmol/l. Presenting clinical features include meconium ileus, malabsorption and steatorrhoea, bronchiectasis, intrahepatic cholestasis and gallstones, delayed puberty and maturity, diabetes mellitus, and altered fertility.

72. FTTTT

An intra-operative transfusion reaction is characterized by hypotension, fever and increased bleeding at the operative site. If the operation is performed under regional anaesthesia the patient may also complain of pruritus and dyspnoea.

73. **Regarding sickle-cell anaemia**
    A. It results from a point mutation in the sixth codon of the beta globin gene, leading to substitution of glutamic acid for valine
    B. Homozygotes have >75% of their haemoglobin as HbS
    C. Deoxygenated HbS tends to form unstable polymers which lead to red cell distortion but normal red cell survival
    D. Parvovirus infection commonly causes acute haemolytic crises
    E. Dactylitis is not uncommon in children with sickle-cell disease

74. **The fat embolus syndrome**
    A. Arises in 3% of patients following hip surgery
    B. Classically there is a triad of respiratory insufficiency, mental changes and low grade pyrexia
    C. The mental changes are mild and self-limiting
    D. During surgery on the femur, intramedullary pressures may rise to 30–40 mmHg
    E. ARDS may result

75. **Regarding hypothermia**
    A. Less oxygen is dissolved in the plasma of hypothermic patients
    B. Coagulation occurs more rapidly due to increased blood viscosity and a reduction in blood flow
    C. The heart rate is maintained until core temperature falls to 25°C
    D. Bronchoconstriction is associated with hypothermia
    E. At 25°C the brain can remain ischaemic for approximately 45 min before cerebral damage occurs

73. FTFTT

In sickle-cell anaemia there is substitution of valine for glutamic acid and not vice versa. Red blood cell survival is shortened in this disease. A definition always gets the question off to a good start. The 'anaesthetic implications of the disease' is a bread-and-butter topic in the FRCA exam and a good one in which to score well.

74. FFFFT

The incidence of fat embolus syndrome after hip surgery is 0.1%. The classic triad of clinical features is respiratory insufficiency, mental changes and petechial haemorrhages. The mental changes may be severe and can include convulsions and coma. The normal femoral intramedullary pressures are 30–40 mmHg. During surgery on the femur these may rise to 1400 mmHg. Lung damage by fat emboli may lead to ARDS.

75. FFFFF

Solubility increases as temperature falls. 0.3 ml/dl of oxygen is dissolved in the blood of normothermic patients, whereas at 10°C 3.2 ml/dl will be dissolved. The oxygen dissociation curve will also be shifted to the left in hypothermia (the Bohr effect). Coagulation slows in hypothermia due to the inhibition of enzymes. The heart rate slows linearly with temperature due to a direct effect on the sinoatrial node. In the healthy, well-perfused heart, asystole occurs at 20°C. However, ventricular fibrillation can occur at temperatures as high as 32°C if there is myocardial hypoxia, poor coronary perfusion or electrolyte and acid–base disturbances. The bronchioles dilate in hypothermic patients. The brain can remain ischaemic for only 15 min at 25°C before cerebral damage occurs.

76. Useful strategies to prevent airway fires include
   A.   Filling the endotracheal tube cuff with saline
   B.   Avoidance of red rubber tubes
   C.   Limiting inspired oxygen and increasing inspired nitrous oxide
   D.   Using helium as the carrier gas
   E.   Wrapping the endotracheal tube in moistened muslin

77. Regarding antibiotics
   A.   Ciprofloxacin is only effective against Gram-positive bacteria
   B.   Imipenem is a β-lactam antibiotic
   C.   Vancomycin is an aminoglycoside
   D.   Metronidazole may cause peripheral neuropathy following prolonged therapy
   E.   Ceftazidime is effective against pseudomonas

78. Recognized effects of permissive hypercapnia include
   A.   Increased cardiac output
   B.   Reduced systemic vascular resistance
   C.   Reduced pulmonary vascular resistance
   D.   Increased P_aO_2
   E.   Leftward shift of the haemoglobin dissociation curve

76. TFFTF

Filling the endotracheal tube cuff with saline makes perforation by the laser obvious so that remedial action can be taken to prevent leakage of anaesthetic gases into the surgical field. Red rubber tubes have been shown to be more resistant to ignition by the CO_2 laser than PVC tubes. Using nitrous oxide as the carrier gas is as dangerous as using 100% oxygen. Helium has been suggested to be useful as it has a high thermal conductivity and may delay ignition. Additionally, its low density permits the use of smaller endotracheal tubes. Moistened muslin is not useful because it becomes flammable if it dries out during the procedure.

77. FTFTT

Ciprofloxacin is effective against Gram-positive bacteria but is especially useful in the treatment of infections caused by Gram-negative bacteria, e.g. *Pseudomonas*, *Salmonella* and *Neisseria*. β-lactam antibiotics are bactericidal, inhibiting cell wall synthesis. They include penicillins, cephalosporins, aztreonam and imipenem. Vancomycin is not an aminoglycoside and is active against Gram-positive cocci, including multiresistant *Staphylococci*. Ceftazidime is a third-generation cephalosporin with a good effect against Gram-negative organisms, in particular *Pseudomonas*.

78. TTFFF

Permissive hypercapnia by definition results in an increased P_aCO_2. Direct and indirect effects (by sympathetic stimulation) lead to an increased cardiac output, reduced systemic vascular resistance and increased pulmonary vascular resistance. P_aO_2 decreases and the haemoglobin dissociation curve is shifted to the right.

79. In pleural effusion
   A. Left ventricular failure accounts for 40% of effusions
   B. A protein content of >30 g/l is diagnostic of a transudate
   C. A blood-stained transudate is common in bronchial carcinoma or metastatic breast carcinoma
   D. Acute pancreatitis commonly causes a left-sided transudate
   E. The glucose level is high when rheumatoid arthritis is the cause

80. Anaesthesia and the liver
   A. Regional anaesthesia maintains liver blood flow
   B. IPPV reduces liver blood flow
   C. Volatile anaesthetics increase liver blood flow
   D. Halothane is 10% liver metabolized
   E. Reductive metabolites of halothane are causative in halothane hepatitis

81. The following are absolute indications for a double lumen tube
   A. Resection of a bronchopleural fistula
   B. Drainage of a lung abscess
   C. Resection of a giant air cyst
   D. Pneumonectomy
   E. Resection of a thoracic artery aneurysm

79. TFFFF
Pleural effusion is commonly caused by left ventricular failure. Other main causes include bacterial pneumonia (24%), malignancy (15%), viral infections (8%), pulmonary embolism (6%) and cirrhosis (4%). The protein content differentiates a transudate (<30 g/l) from an exudate (>30 g/l). Cardiac failure, nephrotic syndrome, myxoedema, constrictive pericarditis and Meig's syndrome cause transudates. Exudates are caused by bacterial pneumonia, carcinoma and pleural inflammation which is caused by pulmonary infarction and tuberculosis, autoimmune rheumatic disease, acute pancreatitis and subphrenic or hepatic abscess. The glucose content is low in rheumatoid arthritis, tuberculosis and carcinoma.

80. FTFFF
Regional anaesthesia depresses liver blood flow in proportion to the reduction in mean arterial pressure. Both IPPV and volatile anaesthetics depress liver blood flow secondary to a reduction in cardiac output. Halothane is 20% liver-metabolized. Liver damage secondary to halothane anaesthesia is now considered to be related to trifluoroacetyl halide, an oxidative metabolite of halothane.

81. TTTFF
Absolute indications for a double lumen tube (DLT) include isolation to prevent spillage of infected material into the non-infected lung, such as may result from surgery involving a lung abscess or bronchopleural fistula. In the absence of a DLT a giant air cyst may rupture causing a tension pneumothorax with IPPV. Pneumonectomy and resection of a thoracic aortic aneurysm are not absolute indications.

82. **The following drugs are safe to use in patients with malignant hyperpyrexia**
    A. Sevoflurane
    B. Alfentanil
    C. Propofol
    D. Nitrous oxide
    E. Suxamethonium

83. **Regarding magnesium**
    A. Magnesium is largely an extracellular ion
    B. The normal plasma concentration of magnesium is 0.75–1.05 mmol/l
    C. Hypomagnesaemia is associated with hypophosphataemia
    D. Hypomagnesaemia potentiates non-depolarizing neuromuscular blockade
    E. Magnesium has no effect on uterine contraction

84. **Barotrauma**
    A. Pulmonary interstitial emphysema is not visible on chest X-ray
    B. Pneumothorax generally precedes the development of mediastinal emphysema
    C. May lead to pneumo-retroperitoneum
    D. Development is associated with decreased intravascular pressures
    E. Is more common in compliant lungs

82. FTTTF
If you know the list of safe drugs you will be OK both in MCQs and when it comes to anaesthetizing these challenging patients! Definite triggers of malignant hyperpyrexia are the volatile anaesthetic agents and suxamethonium. All local anaesthetic agents are considered to be as safe as each other. Propofol is safe to use.

83. FTTFF
Magnesium is largely an intracellular ion with 50% of total magnesium in bone. Hypomagnesaemia, as well as hyperparathyroidism, alkalosis and haemodialysis, causes hypophosphataemia. Hypermagnesaemia potentiates neuromuscular blockade by decreasing acetylcholine release and reducing the sensitivity of the muscle end plate to acetylcholine. Magnesium sulphate has been used as a tocolytic drug.

84. FFTTF
Pulmonary interstitial emphysema (PIE) may be visible on chest X-ray as perivascular collections or subpleural blebs. Air derived from PIE will track towards the hilar regions to form mediastinal emphysema. It may track out of the mediastinum to form a pneumothorax. It may also track along the aorta forming a pneumo-retroperitoneum. Alveolar rupture is more likely to occur if there is an increased pressure gradient between the alveolus and the perivascular tissues. This pressure gradient is increased when the intravascular pressure is low. Barotrauma is a higher risk in poorly compliant lungs.

85. Regarding aortic valve disease
A. The causes of aortic stenosis include a bicuspid aortic valve, ankylosing spondylitis and syphilitic aortitis
B. The three cardinal symptoms of aortic stenosis are angina, breathlessness and dizziness or syncope on exercise
C. Signs of aortic regurgitation are a collapsing pulse and an ejection systolic murmur with a palpable ejection systolic thrill
D. A gradient across the valve of 30 mmHg is indicative of severe aortic stenosis
E. The electrocardiograph in aortic stenosis shows left ventricular hypertrophy and a strain pattern of pressure overload

86. The following statements regarding statistics are true
A. The median of a population equals the mean for a normal distribution
B. The mode of a set of observations is the value with an equal number of values above and below it
C. The mode of a population equals the mean for a normal distribution
D. Standard error = standard deviation $\div n$ (where n = number of values)
E. Standard deviation = $\sqrt{\text{variance}}$

85. FTFFT

The causes of aortic stenosis are congenital (bicuspid valve), rheumatoid arthritis and senile calcification of the valve leaflets. The causes listed in this part of the question are those of aortic regurgitation. Patients with aortic regurgitation have an early diastolic murmur. If ventricular function is normal, a gradient of 30 mmHg is considered mild aortic stenosis, a gradient of 30–70 mmHg is indicative of moderate stenosis and a gradient of >70 mmHg is considered severe. If left ventricular function is poor and cardiac output is reduced then the gradient is less for each category. The ECG in aortic stenosis shows left ventricular hypertrophy and a strain pattern of pressure overload, i.e. depressed ST segments, T wave inversion and increased voltages in the left ventricular leads.

86. TFTFT

Median describes the middle value of a set of observations or measurements. It is the value on the fiftieth percentile with an equal number of measurements above and below it. The mean of a set of observations is the sum of their values divided by the number of observations. Therefore for a normal distribution the median is the same as the mean. The mode is the value in a set of observations which occurs most often and may be to the left or the right of the mean but in a normal distribution will equal the mean and the median. Standard error describes how well the sample mean represents the population mean and how likely it is that the two experimental samples come from the same population. Standard error = standard deviation $\div \sqrt{n}$ (where n = number of values).

87. **Regarding blood products**
    A. Perfluorocarbons are molecules which, when in solution, dissolve oxygen
    B. Platelets can only be stored for 10 days before platelet damage occurs
    C. In an adult, one unit of platelet concentrate raises the platelet count by $5 \times 10^9 \, l^{-1}$
    D. Cryoprecipitate contains thrombin, fibrinogen and factor VIII
    E. Plasma protein fraction (PPF) is rich in coagulation factors II, V, VII, IX and X

88. **The following agents inhibit hypoxic pulmonary vasoconstriction**
    A. Etomidate
    B. Ketamine
    C. Dobutamine
    D. Sodium nitroprusside
    E. Nitrous oxide

89. **Concerning gastric acid secretion**
    A. Gastric acid is required for the absorption of iron
    B. Sucralfate acts predominantly as an antacid
    C. Omeprazole reduces the secretion of hydrochloric acid by blocking the effect of gastrin on the parietal cells of the stomach
    D. Omeprazole prolongs the effect of diazepam and phenytoin
    E. NSAIDs increase gastric acid secretion

87. **TFTFF**
Perfluorocarbons contain 6–10 carbon atoms combined with fluorine and obey Henry's law in dissolving oxygen in solution. They are non-toxic and are used as synthetic haemoglobin substitutes. Platelet concentrates are stored at 20–24°C with continual gentle mixing for up to 5 days. Although after 5 days platelet concentrate maintains clinically useful activity, platelet function deteriorates after 48 h storage. Cryoprecipitate is the precipitate formed when snap-frozen plasma is thawed and contains fibrinogen, fibronectin and factor VIII in a volume of 20 ml. PPF is prepared from plasma which has not been snap-frozen to preserve coagulation factors. It therefore has no coagulation activity.

88. **FFTTT**
Intravenous anaesthetic agents do not inhibit hypoxic pulmonary vasoconstriction. Vasodilator drugs that have been shown to inhibit hypoxic pulmonary vasoconstriction include dobutamine and sodium nitroprusside. Nitrous oxide causes a small but consistent inhibition of hypoxic pulmonary vasoconstriction.

89. **TFFTF**
Gastric acid reduces iron from the Fe^{3+} to the Fe^{2+} form in which it is absorbed. Sucralfate is an aluminium salt of sucrose. It may work by increasing mucosal blood flow and by stimulating the release of protective substances such as prostaglandin E_2 from the gastric mucosa. Sucralfate has little or no antacid activity. Omeprazole inhibits the H^+,K^+-ATPase enzyme which exchanges H^+ and K^+ ions. Diazepam and phenytoin are metabolized in the liver by the cytochrome P_{450} enzyme subset IIC, which is inhibited by omeprazole. NSAIDs inhibit gastric mucosal prostaglandin synthesis, which is needed for the production of the mucous coat that protects the gastric mucosa from gastric acid.

90. Post-herpetic neuralgia
   A. Most commonly involves the lumbar dermatomes
   B. Usually involves multiple dermatomes
   C. The clinical course is characterized by gradual improvement
   D. Tricyclics are beneficial
   E. Morphine is not effective

90. FFTTF

Post-herpetic neuralgia most commonly involves the thoracic dermatomes and the ophthalmic division of the trigeminal nerve. It is usually confined to a single dermatome. The clinical course is one of gradual improvement. Both tricyclics and morphine have been shown to be useful.

Paper 2

1. **The adult respiratory distress syndrome**
   A. Is associated with reduced lung compliance
   B. Both inhaled and intravenous prostacyclin reduce shunt fraction
   C. High-dose steroids are a useful treatment
   D. A pulmonary capillary wedge pressure of 15 mmHg aids diagnosis
   E. The mortality of adult respiratory distress syndrome caused by fat embolus syndrome is 10%

2. **Regarding the treatment of diabetes mellitus**
   A. Velosulin has a peak effect at 6–8 h
   B. Glicazide has a shorter duration of action than glipazide
   C. Biguanides reduce intestinal glucose absorption and stimulate β islet cells to secrete insulin
   D. Aspirin enhances the activity of the sulphonylureas
   E. The duration of action of metformin is 12–18 h

3. **Concerning the measurement of renal function**
   A. Plasma creatinine concentration accurately reflects creatinine clearance by the kidney
   B. Normal creatinine clearance = 125 ml/h
   C. Creatinine clearance overestimates the glomerular filtration rate (GFR)
   D. Cimetidine causes a fall in creatinine clearance
   E. GFR falls in hypothermic patients

1. TFFTT
Adult respiratory distress syndrome (ARDS) is associated with reduced lung compliance. Inhaled prostacyclin lowers the shunt fraction while intravenous prostacyclin increases the shunt fraction. High-dose steroids have not been shown to be of use. Diagnostic criteria for the diagnosis of ARDS include a pulmonary wedge pressure of 15 mmHg or less. The mortality of ARDS associated with fat embolus syndrome is 10%.

2. FFFTF
Velosulin is a short-acting insulin with a peak effect at 2–3 h. Glicazide has a duration of action of 12–18 h whilst glipazide has a duration of action of 6–10 h. Both are sulphonylureas. Biguanides reduce intestinal glucose absorption and enhance insulin sensitivity. It is the sulphonylureas, however, that stimulate β islet cells to secrete insulin. Aspirin displaces sulphonylureas from plasma proteins, thus enhancing their action. The duration of action of metformin is 3–6 h.

3. FFTTT
Plasma creatinine does not accurately reflect creatinine clearance in all clinical situations; in particular, when GFR begins to fall, the initial rise in creatinine concentration is small. Normal creatinine clearance is 125 ml/min. As creatinine is secreted by the distal tubular cells, creatinine clearance overestimates GFR by about 10%. Cimetidine and trimethoprim inhibit creatinine secretion by the distal nephron, leading to a fall in creatinine clearance. Cardiac output, renal blood flow and thus GFR are reduced in hypothermic patients.

4. The Lambert–Eaton myasthenic syndrome
  A. There is reduced sensitivity to non-depolarizing neuromuscular blockers
  B. There is increased sensitivity to depolarizing neuromuscular blockers
  C. The condition is antagonized by 3,4-diaminopyridine
  D. EMG changes are typically mild
  E. Dry mouth is a feature

5. The following drugs may be safely used in the porphyrias
  A. Neostigmine
  B. Pentazocine
  C. Etomidate
  D. Griseofulvin
  E. Droperidol

6. Reflex sympathetic dystrophy
  A. Is associated with myocardial infarction
  B. The skin temperature is lower than normal
  C. The skin temperature is higher than normal
  D. Oedema of the affected area is present
  E. Raised white blood cell count is a feature

7. Regarding tetanus
  A. *Clostridia* are anaerobic, Gram-positive, spore-forming bacilli
  B. The exotoxin produced is called tetanospasmin
  C. It affects the posterior horns of the spinal cord and medulla, where the normal inhibitory input to the motor neurones is blocked
  D. The incubation period is 12 h
  E. Clinical features include muscular rigidity and spasms, together with a decreased level of consciousness

4. **FTTFT**
   The Lambert–Eaton myasthenic syndrome is due to decreased quantal release of acetylcholine, resulting in increased sensitivity to both depolarizing and non-depolarizing neuromuscular blockers. Although clinical features may not be severe, EMG changes are typically marked. Acetylcholine release may also be reduced at cholinergic autonomic sites, which is manifested as dry mouth, blurred vision or constipation.

5. **TFFFT**
   Pentazocine, etomidate, griseofulvin, alcohol, thiopentone, the contraceptive pill, prochlorperazine, sulphonamides, alpha methyl-dopa and flunitrazepam are unsafe in the presence of porphyria.

6. **TTTTF**
   Reflex sympathetic dystrophy is most commonly precipitated by trauma. However, it may have other precipitating causes including myocardial infarction. Reflex sympathetic dystrophy evolves through three stages. During stage one the skin is warm, during stages two and three it becomes cool. Oedema is a feature of reflex sympathetic dystrophy. Raised white cell count is not a feature.

7. **TTFFF**
   Tetanus affects the anterior horns of the spinal cord. The incubation period is variable and ranges from some days to months. The level of consciousness is normal with the disease but severe illness can be accompanied by marked autonomic changes.

8. The following drugs increase gastric emptying
  A. Atropine
  B. Metoclopramide
  C. Cisapride
  D. Carbenoxolone
  E. Ephedrine

9. Regarding pH
  A. The pH of a 1 molar solution of hydrochloric acid (HCl) is 1
  B. A litre solution, the pH of which is 2.4, contains $10^{-2.4}$ g of H^+ ions
  C. When fully dissociated, pure water contains H^+ and OH^- ions in equal proportions
  D. There is a linear relationship between pH and PCO_2 in the blood
  E. The pH of compound sodium lactate solution (Hartmann's solution) is 5

10. The neonatal airway
  A. The larynx lies opposite C4–C5
  B. The trachea is 3–4 cm long
  C. The tracheal rings are fully developed
  D. The nasal passages account for up to 40% of the total airway resistance
  E. The cricoid cartilage is the narrowest part of the airway

8. FTTFF

Drugs that promote the release of acetylcholine in the myenteric plexus are prokinetic. Atropine, therefore, not only reduces gastric motility but also reduces gastric acid secretion by half. Metoclopramide is a D_2 antagonist, although this is probably not how it promotes gastric emptying. It either stimulates the release of acetylcholine in the myenteric plexus or mediates its action through the 5-HT_4 receptor in the gut wall. Cisapride is chemically related to metoclopramide and acts in a similar way to increase gastric emptying; however, it has no anti-dopaminergic and thus no central anti-emetic effects. Carbenoxolone is a synthetic derivative of a component of liquorice. It has no effect on gastric emptying but does have a protective effect on gastric mucosa, due to an increased level of prostaglandins, and an effect on nitric oxide.

9. FTTFF

Sørensen introduced the concept of pH to express in logarithmic terms the hydrogen ion concentration of a solution. The letter p stands for 'Potenz' or 'Power' and $C_H = 10^{-p}$, where C_H is the hydrogen ion concentration. As the hydrogen ion concentration (C_H) of a 1 M HCl solution is 1 g/l, the pH is 0 (as $10^0 = 1$). Similarly, a solution with a pH of 2.4 contains $10^{-2.4}$ g/l of H^+ ions. When fully dissociated, a litre of water contains 10^{-7} OH^- ions and 10^{-7} H^+ ions and therefore has a pH of 7. There is a semi-logarithmic relationship between pH and PCO_2 in the blood. The pH of Hartmann's solution is 6.

10. FFFFT

The full term neonatal larynx lies opposite C3–C4. The trachea is 4–5 cm long with tracheal rings that are incompletely developed and non-calcified. The nasal passages account for >50% of airway resistance.

11. Bronchial carcinoma
A. May present with atrial fibrillation
B. May cause diaphragmatic paralysis
C. Presents with local symptoms in 25% of patients, metastases in 65% of patients and non-metastatic manifestations in the remaining 10%
D. May cause Addison's disease
E. May present with hypercalcaemia

12. Nosocomial pneumonia in the ITU
A. Causative organisms are usually of exogenous origin
B. Causative organisms are usually Gram-positive
C. SPEAR has been shown to lower overall mortality
D. *Pseudomonas* is commonly implicated
E. Mortality is approximately 30%

13. Regarding pericardial disease
A. Acute pericarditis most commonly follows myocardial infarction
B. The electrocardiogram in acute pericarditis shows upwardly concave ST-segment depression in all leads
C. The electrocardiogram in pericardial effusion shows reduced voltages with electrical alternans
D. In healthy patients the two layers of visceral pericardium normally contain up to 15 ml of fluid
E. Signs of cardiac tamponade include a paradoxical pulse and a positive Kussmaul's sign

14. The following physiological variables are measured in the APACHE II scoring system
A. Arterial pH
B. Serum potassium
C. Glasgow coma score
D. Central venous pressure
E. Blood glucose

11. **TTFTT**
Atrial fibrillation can be caused as a direct result of invasion of the pericardium by the tumour. Tumours at either hilum can cause phrenic nerve palsies. Presentation with local symptoms occurs in 75% of patients, 13% present with metastases and 12% with non-metastatic manifestations. Adrenal metastases can cause Addison's disease. Non-metastatic manifestations are cutaneous, endocrine, neuromuscular and haematological.

12. **FFFTF**
The causative organisms of nosocomial pneumonia are usually endogenous Gram-negative aerobic organisms. *Pseudomonas* is commonly implicated. Selective parenteral and enteral antisepsis regimen (SPEAR) has not been shown to lower overall mortality. The mortality rate associated with nosocomial pneumonia is of the order of 60%.

13. **FFTFT**
The most common cause of acute pericarditis is following coxsackie viral infection, which can be epidemic. Other causes include myocardial infarction, uraemia, connective tissue diseases, post-pericardiotomy, trauma, tuberculosis and neoplasia. The ST segment is elevated in all leads. The visceral pericardium contains at most a few millilitres of fluid. Kussmaul's sign is a raised venous pressure on inspiration, which is abnormal.

14. **TTTFF**
Blood glucose and central venous pressure do not feature in the APACHE II scoring system.

15. The liver is responsible for the production of the following
   A. Bilirubin
   B. Prealbumin
   C. Fibrinogen
   D. Urea
   E. Factor VIII

16. Duchenne's muscular dystrophy
   A. Pre-operative pulmonary function tests show an obstructive picture
   B. Patients are at risk of aspiration
   C. A resting tachycardia is innocent
   D. A pre-operative echocardiogram is useful
   E. Suxamethonium does not cause hyperkalaemia if the condition is not clinically manifest

17. Thrombosis is predisposed by
   A. Inherited disorders of Protein C
   B. Inherited disorders of Protein S
   C. Antithrombin III
   D. Lupus anticoagulant
   E. Inherited disorders of tissue plasminogen activator

15. **FTTTF**

Bilirubin is formed in the tissues from the breakdown of haemoglobin. Free bilirubin is conjugated with glucuronic acid in the liver. Albumin is produced by the liver and is responsible for the maintenance of oncotic pressure and the transport of many substances in the blood, e.g. bilirubin, drugs, trace metals and fatty acids. Albumin has a half-life of 20 days. The liver also produces prealbumin which, as it has a half-life of 1.5 days, is a more useful marker of liver disease than albumin. The liver produces fibrinogen, prothrombin and clotting factors V, VII, IX and X. Most of the amino acids entering the liver, except for the branch-chained amino acids leucine, isoleucine and valine, are catabolized to urea.

16. **FTFTF**

Pulmonary function tests show a restrictive picture. Poor oesophageal motility and delayed gastric emptying increase the risk of aspiration. Cardiomyopathy is a constant feature. It is often manifest by a resting tachycardia. Mitral regurgitation secondary to papillary muscle dysfunction is also a feature and therefore echocardiography is useful. Suxamethonium has caused hyperkalaemia in both recognized and unrecognized cases.

17. **TTFTT**

The aetiology of thrombosis is either inherited or acquired. The inherited diseases are given in the question. In addition, antithrombin III deficiency causes thrombosis. Acquired risk factors include lupus anticoagulant, immobility, obesity, the puerperium, the contraceptive pill, some surgery, smoking, burns and autoimmune disorders. Inherited thrombophilias have a prevalence of 1:7500.

18. Markers of severity in acute pancreatitis include
   A.   Age <50 years
   B.   White cell count >16 × 10^9/l
   C.   Hypocalcaemia
   D.   Hypoxaemia
   E.   Renal impairment (urea rise >2 mmol/l)

19. Helium and oxygen mixtures
   A.   Cylinders have a brown body with a black-and-white quartered shoulder
   B.   Cylinders have a pressure of 54 bar
   C.   Reduce the work of breathing at turbulent flows
   D.   Are useful in both upper and lower airway obstructions
   E.   Are less viscous than air

20. The following criteria should be met prior to weaning from mechanical ventilation
   A.   Phosphate levels should be of the order of 1.0 mmol/l
   B.   Discontinuation of inotropic support
   C.   Ability to generate an inspiratory force of −10 cmH$_2$O
   D.   Vital capacity of 10–15 ml/kg
   E.   Minute ventilation above 10 l/min

18. **FTFTT**
    Markers of the severity of acute pancreatitis are age >55 years, a white cell count >16 × 10⁹/l, hypocalcaemia <2 mmol/l, hypoxaemia <8 kPa and an acidosis with a base deficit >4 mmol/l. Acute pancreatitis is a relatively common condition presenting to the ITU. The commonest causes in the UK are gallstones and alcohol. Complications are classified into local (pseudocyst, gastrointestinal bleeding, ileus) or systemic (respiratory failure, acute renal failure, hyperglycaemia, hypocalcaemia, DIC) and may be early or late.

19. **FFTFF**
    Helium (79%) and oxygen (21%) mixtures are supplied in cylinders which have a brown body and a white and brown shoulder. They are pressurized to 137 bar. Helium and oxygen mixtures are less dense than air, thus reducing the tendency to turbulent flow (lowering Reynold's number). The work of breathing is therefore reduced. Turbulent flow occurs in upper, not lower airway obstruction. In lower airway obstruction the flow remains laminar. As helium and oxygen mixtures are more viscous than air they are not useful in lower airway obstruction.

20. **TFFTF**
    There have been a number of suggested criteria that should be present prior to weaning from mechanical ventilation. As hypophosphataemia contributes to muscle weakness it should be normalized (0.8–1.45 mmol/l). Weaning may proceed in the presence of inotropic support. The ability to generate a negative inspiratory pressure of −20 cmH₂O, a vital capacity of 10–15 ml/kg and a minute ventilation <10 l/min are all recognized criteria.

21. **Regarding mitral valve disease**
    A. The main cause of mitral stenosis in the UK is congenital and is associated with abnormalities of the left ventricle
    B. Collagen disorders can cause mitral regurgitation
    C. In mitral stenosis, auscultation of the heart reveals a mid-diastolic murmur, a loud first heart sound and an opening snap which is heard in early diastole
    D. Prophylaxis against thromboembolism with warfarin is essential and should be started early and not only when atrial fibrillation has developed
    E. Treatment of mitral regurgitation includes vasodilators, such as ACE inhibitors, which act by encouraging forward flow from the left ventricle

22. **Regarding anti-emetic drugs**
    A. Hyoscine is of little benefit in the treatment of motion sickness
    B. Droperidol and prochlorperazine have marked affinity for central dopamine receptors
    C. Cyclizine should be avoided in patients with porphyria
    D. Metoclopramide increases lower oesophageal sphincter tone
    E. Droperidol causes hypotension in some patients

21. FTTTT

The main cause of mitral stenosis is rheumatic fever. It is rarely congenital, and signs of stenosis occur with SLE, senile calcification of the valve ring and infective endocarditis with fleshy vegetations. The causes of mitral incompetence are mitral valve prolapse, rheumatic heart disease, left ventricular dilatation (cardiomyopathy), ischaemic heart disease with papillary muscle dysfunction, collagen disorders such as Marfan's syndrome or Ehlers–Danlos syndrome, hypertrophic cardiomyopathy, infective endocarditis and connective tissue disorders such as SLE.

22. FTFTT

Muscarinic receptors are found in the chemoreceptor trigger zone (CTZ). They are also located in the motor nucleus of the vagus nerve and the nucleus ambiguus, which are both involved with vomiting. Hyoscine has marked anticholinergic properties, which account for its antiemetic properties. However, its ability to prevent motion sickness is due to an effect on the vestibular apparatus. Dopamine receptors (D_2) are found in the area postrema that contains the CTZ. Metoclopramide blocks dopamine receptors in the CTZ, hastens gastric emptying and increases lower oesophageal sphincter tone. Droperidol is a D_2 antagonist and also has an α-blocking effect that causes hypotension in some patients.

23. Anaesthesia and ECT
- A. Emergence phenomena are common when ketamine is used
- B. An immediate tachycardia followed by a bradycardia is the norm
- C. Lithium should be continued up to the time of ECT
- D. A myocardial infarct within the past 3 months is a relative contraindication
- E. Pregnancy is an absolute contraindication

24. Disseminated intravascular coagulation (DIC) occurs in the following conditions
- A. Gram-positive infections
- B. Amniotic fluid embolism
- C. Intrauterine death
- D. Incompatible blood transfusion
- E. Anaphylaxis

25. Persistent hypophosphataemia causes
- A. Haemolysis
- B. Reduced oxygen delivery
- C. Osborn waves on the ECG
- D. Paraesthesia
- E. Increased platelet aggregation

23. FFFFF

When ketamine has been used for ECT, emergence phenomena have been reported to be comparatively rare when compared to other applications of ketamine. ECT results in immediate parasympathetic activation followed by sympathetic activation. Although a variety of arrhythmias may occur, a bradycardia followed by a tachycardia is the most common. Lithium increases post-ECT confusion and should be withheld prior to ECT. With regard to contraindications, the risk of ECT must be weighed against the risks of ECT being withheld. However, a myocardial infarct occurring within the past 3 months is recognized as an absolute contraindication while pregnancy is a relative contraindication.

24. TTTTT

Gram-negative infections are normally associated with DIC, although any infection can cause it. The causes are classified into infections (Gram-negative, meningococcal, clostridial or viral), malignancy (solid tumours, leukaemia), obstetric (amniotic fluid embolus, IUD, PET, retained placenta), immunological (anaphylaxis, incompatible blood transfusion), liver disease (acute liver failure, cirrhosis, Reye's syndrome) and snake bites.

25. TTFTF

Prolonged hypophosphataemia causes a reduction in ATP within red cells, white cells and platelets leading to haemolysis, reduced neutrophil function and impaired platelet aggregation. A reduction in 2,3 DPG causes reduced oxygen delivery by shifting the oxygen dissociation curve to the left. Hypophosphataemia also causes weakness, hypotension, heart failure, paraesthesia and respiratory muscle weakness. The Osborn wave is an upward deflection on the downstroke of the R wave and is found in patients with moderate hypothermia.

26. Concerning electricity and electrical circuits
  A. The volt is the SI unit of potential difference and is the work done in moving a unit charge from one point to another
  B. The heat generated when a current flows through a resistance is proportional to the square of the resistance
  C. For resistances occurring in parallel in an electrical circuit, the net resistance is less than the smallest of the individual resistances
  D. 1 ampere = 1 coulomb/second
  E. A capacitor conducts direct current (dc) but does not conduct alternating current (ac)

27. The following are all forms of sterilization
  A. Soaking for 30 min in 0.05% chlorhexidine
  B. Applying dry heat at 160°C for 20–30 min
  C. Pasteurization
  D. Boiling for 5 min
  E. Autoclaving

28. Regarding α_1-antitrypsin deficiency
  A. It has an autosomal recessive inheritance
  B. α_1 antitrypsin is a protease activator
  C. Reduced protease activity leads to emphysema and chronic liver disease
  D. Chronic liver disease occurs because the hepatocyte fails to excrete α_1 antitrypsin
  E. It may present as neonatal hepatitis or with the complications of cirrhosis

26. TFTTF

Current is the quantity of charge flowing per unit time, i.e. $I = C/s$ (where I is the current in amperes and C is the charge in coulombs). As $P = I^2R$ (where P is power, or heat generated, in watts and I is the current flowing through a resistance R), heat production is proportional to the square of the current. This principle is used in diathermy. Resistances in series are additive. However, for resistances in parallel the current from the battery is the sum of the currents flowing through each parallel branch, i.e. $I = I_1 + I_2 + I_3 + I_n = V(1/R_1 + 1/R_2 + 1/R_3 + 1/R_n) = V/R_p$ Therefore, $1/R_p = 1/R_1 + 1/R_2 + 1/R_3 + 1/R_n$ R_p, the net resistance, is thus smaller than the smallest of the parallel resistances. A capacitor accumulates charge but does not conduct direct current. The charge it accumulates is proportional to the potential difference applied across it. The SI unit is the coulomb per volt, or farad. Capacitors do conduct ac current.

27. FTFFT

Autoclaving and applying dry heat at $160°C$ for 20–30 min are both examples of sterilization. The remainder are examples of disinfection.

28. FFFTT

α_1 antitrypsin deficiency is normally associated in the anaesthetist's mind with emphysema and the anaesthetic implications of chronic lung disease. α_1 antitrypsin is a protease inhibitor and it is the unchecked protease activity that accounts for the emphysema and chronic liver disease. The disease is inherited as an autosomal dominant condition. The diagnosis can be made by measuring serum levels, but these are not always low and confirmation is made by measuring the phenotype.

29. Antidotes to cyanide poisoning
- A. Sodium thiosulphate has a rapid onset
- B. Sodium thiosulphate transfers sulphur to cyanide
- C. Dicobalt edetate converts cyanide to a renally excreted compound
- D. Dicobalt edetate should be administered in saline
- E. Nitrites may aggravate hypoxia

30. The following statements about endotoxin are true
- A. It is situated on the outer membrane of Gram-negative organisms
- B. 'A' antigens are used for typing bacteria
- C. 'O' antigens are made up of lipid
- D. Endotoxin stimulates the release of TNF from macrophages
- E. 'R' antigen consists of glycolipid

31. The following drugs increase respiratory drive
- A. Acetazolamide
- B. Octreotide
- C. Flumazenil
- D. Nikethamide
- E. Doxapram

29. FTTFT
Sodium thiosulphate converts cyanide to thiocyanate. It has a large detoxifying capacity but a slow onset of action. Dicobalt edetate has a rapid onset. It chelates cyanide and produces renally excretable compounds. It may cause hypoglycaemia and should therefore be administered in dextrose. Nitrites produce methaemoglobin, which will combine with cyanide. Methaemoglobinaemia is a cause of hypoxia.

30. TFFTF
Endotoxin is found in the outer membrane of the cell wall of Gram-negative organisms. It consists of three parts:
A surface 'O' antigen consisting of polysaccharide. This antigen is very variable and is used for typing bacterial species.
A core 'R' antigen consisting of oligosaccharides.
An innermost 'A' antigen consisting of lipid. It is structurally highly conserved. Endotoxin stimulates tumour necrosis factor alpha release from macrophages.

31. TFFTT
Acetazolamide, a carbonic anhydrase inhibitor, causes increased excretion of sodium bicarbonate in an alkaline urine and a metabolic acidosis that stimulates respiration. Octreotide is a somatostatin analogue used in the treatment of carcinoid syndrome. Flumazenil reduces the respiratory depressant effects induced by benzodiazepines but has no direct effect on the central nervous system. Nikethamide and doxapram are analeptics which act by stimulating central excitatory pathways. Increased heart rate and arrhythmias occur.

32. **Gas chromatography can be used for measuring the following gases and vapours**
    A. Carbon dioxide
    B. Nitrous oxide
    C. Oxygen
    D. Nitrogen
    E. Halothane

33. **The following increase the risk of spinal haematoma after regional anaesthesia**
    A. Increasing age
    B. Female sex
    C. The presence of an epidural catheter
    D. Spinal abnormalities
    E. Technically difficult needle placement

34. **Symptoms of hypercalcaemia include**
    A. Anorexia
    B. Diarrhoea
    C. Polyuria
    D. Polydypsia
    E. Depression

32. TTTTT

In a gas chromatograph gases pass through a column of polyethylene-coated silica–alumina at different rates depending on their solubility. At the distal end of the chromatograph gases are detected as they emerge from the column. There are three main types of detector. The flame ionization detector is used to detect most organic vapours. The thermal conductivity detector, or katharometer, is used for the analysis of oxygen, nitrogen, carbon dioxide and nitrous oxide. The electron capture detector is used in the analysis of halothane, chloroform, trilene and methoxyflurane.

33. TTTTT

Spinal haematoma following regional anaesthesia has been more commonly reported in elderly females. The type of regional technique is significant, haematomas occurring most commonly with epidural catheters rather than single-shot epidurals or spinal anaesthesia. Spinal abnormalities such as arteriovenous malformations or spina bifida can increase the risk of bleeding. Technically difficult needle placement with multiple attempts increases the risk of haematoma.

34. TFTTT

Symptoms of hypercalcaemia are only likely if the serum calcium level is >3 mmol/l and consist of three major entities: polyuria and polydypsia; nausea, constipation and anorexia; depression and sleep disturbance. Such symptoms may have existed for years prior to diagnosis and it should be remembered that the elderly can present acutely with drowsiness, confusion and dehydration.

35. Salicylate poisoning may result in
A. Respiratory acidosis
B. Coma
C. Increased prothrombin time
D. Thrombocytopenia
E. Death, if blood levels reach 5 mmol/l

36. The following statements regarding diuretics are true
A. Hyponatraemia is more likely in patients taking loop diuretics than thiazide diuretics
B. Amiloride is an aldosterone inhibitor similar to spironolactone
C. Hypokalaemia is more likely in patients taking loop diuretics than thiazide diuretics
D. Frusemide reduces renal blood flow
E. Mannitol has no effect on renal blood flow

37. The occulocardiac reflex
A. Is associated with retrobulbar block
B. Is associated with retrobulbar haemorrhage
C. The afferent limb consists of parasympathetic fibres accompanying the oculomotor nerve
D. The reflex exhibits fatigue
E. The elderly should be given prophylactic anticholinergics

35. **TTTFF**
Salicylate poisoning initially causes a respiratory alkalosis; however, if severe, direct respiratory depression may arise causing a respiratory acidosis. Coma is a feature of severe toxicity. Salicylates cause hepatic damage, as indicated by an increased prothrombin time. Dehydration may lead to an elevated platelet count. Fatalities may arise when plasma levels exceed 7 mmol/l.

36. **FFFFF**
Loop diuretics, unlike thiazides, block the active reabsorption of sodium in the ascending limb of the loop of Henle, thus preventing a rise in interstitial sodium concentration. Therefore, less water is reabsorbed in the collecting ducts of patients taking loop diuretics than those taking thiazide diuretics. While thiazides are less potent than loop diuretics, hyponatraemia is more likely, not because of sodium loss but because of excessive water retention. Spironolactone and amiloride are both potassium-sparing diuretics. Spironolactone inhibits aldosterone whereas amiloride blocks luminal channels, thus preventing transtubular transport of NaCl. Both mannitol and frusemide increase renal blood flow.

37. **TTFTF**
Administration of a retrobulbar block is a known cause of the oculocardiac reflex. Retrobulbar haemorrhage may cause a delayed oculocardiac reflex if sufficient blood is deposited to elevate intraocular pressure. The afferent limb of the reflex is the trigeminal nerve. The reflex fatigues with repeated stimulation. In the elderly the incidence of the reflex is reduced and prophylactic anticholinergics do not offer an advantage.

38. Regarding platelet disorders
   A. Haemostasis usually remains intact unless the platelet count falls below $100 \times 10^9/l$
   B. Chronic idiopathic thrombocytopenia requires low dose steroid (prednisolone 5 mg/day) therapy
   C. Splenectomy is a second-line treatment for chronic idiopathic thrombocytopenia and is 99% effective
   D. Acute thrombocytopenic purpura usually occurs post-virally in children
   E. Infectious mononucleosis causes decreased peripheral destruction of platelets

39. Topical anaesthesia of the airway
   A. Topical anaesthesia of the larynx impairs voluntary motor action
   B. Plasma levels of local anaesthetic are higher following upper rather than lower airway administration
   C. Ten per cent cocaine is the appropriate concentration for nasal anaesthesia
   D. Swallowed cocaine is extensively first-pass metabolized
   E. An appropriate dose of lignocaine is 3 mg/kg

40. Concerning neuromuscular blocking agents
   A. Cisatracurium is four times more potent than atracurium
   B. The dose of doxacurium should be reduced in patients with hepatic impairment
   C. Mivacurium is metabolized by plasma cholinesterase at 75% of the rate at which it metabolizes suxamethonium
   D. Rocuronium is more potent than vecuronium
   E. As 80% of a dose of pipercuronium is deacetylated in the liver, the effects are prolonged in patients with impaired liver function

38. FFFTF
Platelet disorders are either qualitative or quantitative. Haemostasis occurs normally unless the platelet count is $< 40 \times 10^9/l$. In obstetrics, regional blockade is not normally undertaken unless the platelet count is $> 80 \times 10^9/l$, although the trend is important when making this decision. Examination candidates must have an opinion about epidural anaesthesia in patients on aspirin and those on low-dose heparin. High-dose steroids (prednisolone 60–100 mg/day) are used to treat chronic idiopathic purpura. Splenectomy has about an 80% response rate in this condition. Increased peripheral destruction of platelets occurs in glandular fever.

39. FFFFT
Topical anaesthesia of the larynx does not impair voluntary motor function. The lower airway has a higher vascularity and a larger surface area than the upper airway; as a result, plasma levels of local anaesthetic are higher following lower airway administration. Ten per cent cocaine should be avoided due to the unacceptably high incidence of adverse effects. Cocaine is metabolized by plasma cholinesterase and is not subject to a high degree of first-pass metabolism.

40. TFTFF
Cisatracurium is a stereoisomer of atracurium which undergoes Hoffman degradation but is less likely to release amine and has a longer duration of action. Doxacurium t metabolized by the liver but is excreted unchanged in the urine. Therefore, the dose should be modified in patients with renal impairment. Rocuronium is a steroid muscle relaxant with 15% the potency of vecuronium. Pipercuronium is excreted, predominantly unchanged, in the urine so that, in patients with renal impairment, the duration of action is increased despite the fact that the liver becomes a secondary route of elimination in such patients.

41. The femoral nerve
   A.   Is derived from L3, L4 and L5
   B.   Lies within the femoral sheath
   C.   Lies medial to the femoral vein
   D.   Supplies the skin over the lateral malleolus
   E.   Continues down the leg as the common peroneal nerve

42. Regarding motor neurone disease
   A.   It is rare in patients over 50 years of age
   B.   Progressive signs of upper and lower motor neurone dysfunction develop
   C.   Fasciculations are not a feature
   D.   It presents as weakness and wasting of the limbs
   E.   Absent reflexes in the limbs are a feature of the disease

43. Concerning limitations of pulmonary artery occlusion pressure (PAOP)
   A.   Left-to-right shunts cause underestimation of LVEDP
   B.   Tachycardia causes underestimation of LVEDP
   C.   Positioning the pulmonary artery catheter tip in West zone 1 leads to overestimation of LVEDP
   D.   The application of PEEP may lead to overestimation of LVEDP
   E.   Aortic stenosis leads to overestimation of LVEDP

41. FFFFF
The femoral nerve is derived from L2, L3 and L4. It lies
outside the femoral sheath and lateral to the femoral vessels.
Below the ligament the femoral nerve divides into the
terminal branches, including the saphenous nerve which
supplies the skin over the medial malleolus. The common
peroneal nerve is a branch of the sciatic nerve.

42. FTFTF
Motor neurone disease is a rare progressive and untreatable
disease. The incidence rises with age and it is rare in patients
under 50 years. Features include brisk reflexes, even when
the patient has severe wasting. Fasciculation is a feature of
the disease. Apart from the peripheral features of the
disease, bulbar features occur and symptoms include slurred
speech, difficulty in swallowing, a hoarse voice and an
inability to cough. Mental function is preserved even in
severe disease. Treatment is symptomatic.

43. FFTTF
PAOP will overestimate LVEDP when pulmonary blood flow
is increased by left-to-right shunts. Tachycardia limits left
atrial emptying, causing PAOP to overestimate LVEDP.
Positioning the catheter tip in West zone 1 leads to PAOP
reflecting alveolar rather than pulmonary venous pressure. A
similar effect can arise with the application of PEEP. Aortic
stenosis limits ventricular compliance with consequent PAOP
underestimating LVEDP.

44. Regarding the electrocardiogram (ECG)
  A.   J waves are found in patients with hypomagnesaemia
  B.   Right axis deviation is associated with right bundle branch block and left anterior hemiblock
  C.   When recording the ECG, standard lead I records between the left leg and right arm
  D.   The normal P wave is positive in all leads
  E.   The U wave follows the T wave and is more prominent in hypothermic patients

45. Carbon dioxide absorbers
  A.   Both soda lime and baralyme contain silica
  B.   The active carbon dioxide absorber in soda lime is calcium hydroxide
  C.   Barium lime consists of 80% barium hydroxide
  D.   Barium lime is more efficient than soda lime
  E.   The maximum absorption of carbon dioxide by soda lime is 26 l per 100 g

46. Regarding bronchiectasis
  A.   It can occur in children after slowly resolving pneumonias such as after measles
  B.   It is common in patients with IgA deficiency
  C.   Ciliary dysfunction in Kartagener's syndrome occurs
  D.   It is caused by cystic fibrosis as a result of the altered secretions that occur in this disease
  E.   It can be caused by localized bronchial obstruction

44. FFFFF
J waves are positive deflections at the end of the QRS complex and are associated with hypothermia (<30°C). Right axis deviation occurs in right bundle branch block and left posterior hemiblock while right bundle branch block and left axis deviation are associated with left anterior hemiblock. Standard lead I records between the right and left arms. The normal P wave is negative in aVR. The U wave is a positive deflection which follows the T wave made more prominent by hypokalaemia.

45. FFFFT
Barium lime is more stable and does not require the addition of silica. The active component of soda lime for the absorption of carbon dioxide is sodium hydroxide. Barium lime consists of 20% barium hydroxide and 80% calcium hydroxide. Baralyme is 15% less efficient than soda lime.

46. TTTTT
The causes of bronchiectasis can be differentiated into localized bronchial obstruction (inhaled foreign body, enlarged hilar nodes, bronchial tumours) and generalized bronchial obstruction associated with reduced secretion clearance. This occurs in slow-to-resolve pneumonias, recurrent infections in immune defects, altered secretions and ciliary dysfunction. The disease is characterized by chronic cough and copious sputum. The respiratory features are helped diagnostically by the fact that these patients often have finger clubbing. Kartaganer's syndrome is a congenital disease with abnormal cilia and is characterized by bronchiectasis, dextrocardia, sinusitis and male infertility.

47. Platelet-activating factor
A. Is a polypeptide molecule
B. Weakly promotes vascular permeability
C. Activates monocytes, increasing the release of tumour necrosis factor α
D. Is released from platelets
E. Has a positive inotropic effect

48. The following statements regarding the treatment of hypertension are true
A. Enalapril is shorter acting than captopril
B. Captopril prolongs the effect of bradykinin
C. Enalapril has active metabolites
D. Ten per cent of patients taking ACE inhibitors have a positive direct Coombs' test which may interfere with blood cross matching
E. Guanethidine depletes adrenergic neurones of noradrenaline

49. Concerning the mole
A. One mole of gas occupying a volume of 22.4 l exerts a pressure of 1 atm at 273.15 K
B. A mole is the quantity of a substance containing the same number of particles as 12 kg of carbon 12
C. 6.022×10^{23} molecules of hydrogen weighs 1 g
D. 3.4 kg of nitrous oxide occupies 1730 l at standard temperature and pressure (s.t.p.)
E. One mole of solute dissolved in 22.4 l of solution at 0°C exerts an osmotic pressure of 101.3 kPa

50. Protamine
A. Is an acidic molecule
B. Is a protein molecule
C. Has predominantly anti-factor Xa activity
D. Should be given slowly
E. Severe pulmonary hypertension is a direct effect of protamine

47. FFTTF
Platelet-activating factor is a phospholipid. It is a very
potent mediator of increased vascular permeability. Platelet-
activating factor activates monocytes increasing the release
of tumour necrosis factor α. It is released from macrophages,
neutrophils, eosinophils, endothelial cells and platelets.
Tumour necrosis factor α is a negative inotrope.

48. FTTFT
Enalapril has a half-life of up to 35 h due to its active
metabolites while captopril has a half-life of 2 h. ACE
inhibitors prolong the effect of bradykinin as ACE is
responsible for its breakdown. α-methyldopa causes a
positive direct Coombs' test in 10–20% of patients.

49. TFFTT
One mole is 6.022×10^{23} molecules of a substance. One mole
of a gas at s.t.p. occupies 22.4 l. The weight of one mole of a
substance equals its molecular weight. Therefore, one mole
of carbon 12 weighs 12 g and 1 mole of hydrogen molecules
weighs 2 g. 12 kg of carbon 12 = 1000 moles. One mole of
nitrous oxide weighs 44 g as 44 is the molecular weight of
nitrous oxide. Therefore, 3400 g of nitrous oxide at s.t.p.
occupies 22.4 × 3400/44 l, i.e. 1730 l. Osmotic pressure is the
pressure required across a semi-permeable membrane to
counterbalance the effect of dissolved molecules on the other
side of that membrane.

50. FTFTF
Protamine is a highly positively charged basic protein
molecule. The predominant activity of protamine is its
antithrombin effect and it has limited anti-Xa effect. It
should be given slowly to minimize complications such as
hypotension. Severe pulmonary hypertension is mediated by
heparin–protamine complexes.

51. Near drowning
A. In one-third of cases there is no evidence of water aspiration
B. Ventricular fibrillation is the most common arrhythmia
C. Intracranial hypertension is a recognized cause of death
D. Steroids are a useful adjunct to management
E. Alcohol is commonly implicated in the aetiology

52. Regarding humidity
A. The dew point is the temperature at which the relative humidity is 75% and condensation occurs
B. Regnault's hygrometer contains a pointer attached to a hair, the length of which changes with differing humidity
C. The electrical resistance of lithium chloride alters depending on the surrounding humidity
D. The absolute humidity in the upper trachea is the same as that in the alveolus
E. Ten to fifteen per cent of total basal heat loss occurs in the trachea in the humidification of dry inspired gases

53. The following are Vaughan Williams class Ib anti-arrhythmic drugs
A. Quinidine
B. Amiodarone
C. Flecainide
D. Disopyramide
E. Lignocaine

51. FFTFT
Due to laryngospasm 10% of cases do not aspirate water. As part of the diving reflex bradycardia is the most common arrhythmia associated with near drowning. Near drowning leads to hypoxaemia, which may lead to cerebral oedema and intracranial hypertension. Steroids are of no benefit in the management of near drowning. Alcohol is commonly implicated.

52. FFTFT
The dew point is the temperature at which air is saturated with water and condensation occurs. Regnault's hygrometer is a silver tube containing ether through which air is blown to cool it. When condensation occurs on the outside of the hygrometer, the ambient air is 100% saturated with water at that temperature. Using a graph of temperature versus water content of saturated air the absolute humidity, i.e. the amount of water in a given volume, can be determined. The absolute humidity, in fully saturated gas, in the upper trachea is $34\,g/m^3$ while in the alveolus it is $43\,g/m^3$. This is because the warmer the gas the more the water content when fully saturated.

53. FFFFT
Quinidine and disopyramide are in class Ia. Amiodarone is in class III and flecainide is in class Ic. Other drugs in class Ib are mexilitine, phenytoin and tocainamide.

54. Regarding polycythaemia rubra vera
   A. It describes a red cell count $>6.0 \times 10^{12}/1$ in males
   B. It describes a raised PCV level $>45\%$ in females
   C. It describes a raised haemoglobin level $>15.5\,\mathrm{g/dl}$ in females
   D. Nearly 15% of patients present with arterial or venous occlusion
   E. Abnormal platelet function occurs

55. The saturated vapour pressure
   A. Of a liquid increases when a solute is dissolved in it
   B. Is dependent on the ambient temperature
   C. Equals atmospheric pressure at the boiling point of a liquid
   D. Is proportional to atmospheric pressure
   E. Of a liquid is lowered if a gas is dissolved in it

56. Malignant hyperthermia-susceptible individuals
   A. There is an increased risk of sudden death
   B. Triggering agents may not precipitate malignant hyperthermia
   C. Transmission is autosomal recessive
   D. Elevated creatine kinase is uncommon
   E. Ryanodine receptor abnormalities may be present

54. **TTTFT**
    The term describes a raised red cell count ($>5.5 \times 10^{12}/1$ in females), a raised PCV ($>50\%$ in males) and a raised haemoglobin level (>17.5 g/l in males). About 50% of patients present with occlusive problems: coronary, digital, the leg, splenic, hepatic and portal in nature. Neurological features, including dizziness, headaches and lack of concentration, occur. Bruising and bleeding occur from associated platelet problems. About 10% of patients have gout and 15% of patients have pruritus. It causes splenomegaly.

55. **FTTFT**
    Vapour pressure is dependent on ambient temperature and not atmospheric pressure. When a solute is added to a solvent, the larger solute molecules reduce the surface area available to the smaller solvent molecules to evaporate. The solute therefore reduces the vapour pressure of the solvent. This is Raoult's law. Raoult's law applies to all solutions and the substance dissolved in it can be solid, liquid or gas.

56. **TTFFT**
    There is a higher incidence of sudden death in family members of malignant hyperthermia (MH)-susceptible individuals. MH may arise following previous uneventful triggering anaesthetics. Inheritance of MH is autosomal dominant with 70% of cases having elevated creatine kinase. Demonstrable abnormalities in the ryanodine receptor are present in 3–5% of human MH-susceptible cases.

57. Regarding haemochromatosis
   A. Primary haemochromatosis is inherited as an autosomal dominant disease
   B. Primary haemochromatosis usually presents at <30 years of age
   C. Secondary haemochromatosis usually results from repeated blood transfusions
   D. Deposition of iron in the heart leads to arrhythmias and heart failure
   E. In primary haemochromatosis a defect in the enterocyte causes increased iron absorption

58. Regarding the interpretation of hepatitis B serology
   A. Anti-HBsAg indicates that the patient is currently infected with hepatitis B
   B. HBsAg indicates that the patient is currently infected with hepatitis B
   C. HBeAg indicates active viral replication
   D. Anti-HbcAg (IgG) indicates a past history of hepatitis B infection
   E. Anti-HbcAg (IgG) indicates a recent history of hepatitis B infection

57. FFTTT

The prevalence of haemochromatosis is about 0.4%. It usually presents between 40 and 60 years of age. Primary haemochromatosis is inherited as an autosomal recessive disease. It is primary or secondary: secondary is normally associated with excessive blood transfusions, as in patients with thalassaemia or sickle-cell disease. Alcohol excess also causes it. The deposition of iron occurs in the liver (cirrhosis), skin (slate-grey discolouration), pancreas (diabetes), pituitary (impotence), heart (failure and dysrhythmias) and joints (erosive arthropathy).

58. FTTTF

There are three main antigens associated with the virus: surface antigen (HBsAg), core antigen (HBcAg), and e antigen (HBeAg). The interpretation of the findings is as follows. Anti-HBsAg indicates a past history of infection but that the patient is now immune or vaccinated, anti-HbcAg (IgG) indicates a past history of hepatitis B infection, anti-HbcAg (IgM) indicates a recent history of hepatitis B infection, HBsAg present indicates that the patient is currently infected with hepatitis B, HBeAg present indicates active viral replication and anti-HBeAg indicates little viral replication unless infected with a mutant virus. Hepatitis B DNA can be detected and is often the best indicator of infectivity.

59. The osmolarity of plasma
  A. Is approximately 300 mosmol/l
  B. Is related principally to the concentration of plasma proteins
  C. Is greater than the osmolarity of Ringer's lactate solution
  D. Is measured using the principle that the freezing point of water in plasma is related to the plasma osmolarity
  E. Is similar to the osmolarity of glomerular filtrate

60. The following drugs should be avoided in patients taking MAOIs
  A. Pethidine
  B. Alfentanil
  C. Morphine
  D. Ephedrine
  E. Phenylephrine

61. In dysthyroid eye disease the following occur
  A. Lid lag
  B. Upper lid retraction
  C. Asymmetrical exophthalmos
  D. Papilloedema
  E. Ophthalmoplegia

59. TFTTT
Plasma osmolarity is almost solely related to the concentration of plasma electrolytes. Plasma proteins are responsible for only 1 mosmol/l. The osmolarity of Ringer's lactate is equal to the sum of the osmolarities of all the components. As 1 mmol/l has an osmolarity of 1 mosmol/l and the concentration of electrolytes in Ringer's lactate is 278 mmol/l, the osmolarity is 278 mosmol/l. The freezing point of a liquid is depressed when another substance is dissolved in it. The reduction of the freezing point is proportional to the osmolarity of the resulting solution. Thus, the freezing point of water in plasma or urine is related to its osmolarity and is the principle used by the osmometer.

60. TFFTF
This question is an old chestnut! Pethidine is an opioid that should be avoided in patients taking MAOIs. It blocks neural reuptake of serotonin. This interaction causes potentially life-threatening excitatory or depressive reactions. Indirectly acting sympathomimetics such as ephedrine should be avoided as they precipitate hypertensive crises. Phenylephrine, an α_1 agonist, is a safer alternative.

61. TTTTT
Lid lag occurs because the levator palpebrae superioris muscle is partly innervated by the sympathetic nervous system and excess thyroid hormone increases catecholamine sensitivity. Proptosis is the presence of white sclera between the cornea and the lower eyelid with the patient looking straight ahead. Marked proptosis is exophthalmos and it can be asymmetrical. It is caused by an autoimmune inflammatory reaction within the orbital contents. Ophthalmoplegia is caused by weakness of the extraocular muscles due to inflammation.

62. Amniotic fluid embolism
   A. Has a 20% mortality in the first hour
   B. Is often associated with the use of uterine stimulants
   C. Intracranial haemorrhage is a differential diagnosis
   D. Intravenous steroids are useful
   E. Thrombocytopenia is associated

63. Aprotinin
   A. In low doses inhibits plasmin
   B. Has been used in patients with acute pancreatitis
   C. Dosage is measured in kallikrein inhibitor units (KIU)
   D. Is used to treat per-operative hypotension in patients with carcinoid syndrome
   E. In high dose activates trypsin

64. Regarding exponential processes
   A. Exponential processes can be negative or positive
   B. Ninety-three per cent of an exponential process is complete after two half-lives
   C. Thirty-seven per cent of a quantity is used up after one time constant
   D. In the lung, the time constant of expiration is equal to the product of lung compliance and lung resistance
   E. The change in electrical resistance with temperature in a thermistor is exponential

65. Concerning blood products
   A. The haematocrit of packed cells is 0.5
   B. Platelets have a shelf life of 48 h
   C. Platelets should be transfused through a filter
   D. Platelets do not require ABO cross matching
   E. FFP is rich in fibrinogen

62. FFTTT
Amniotic fluid embolism has a 25–50% mortality in the first hour. In recent reviews uterine stimulation was rarely found to be associated with amniotic fluid embolism. As both intracranial haemorrhage and amniotic fluid embolism may present with seizures, intracranial haemorrhage is included in the differential diagnosis. In nearly all survivors of amniotic fluid embolism intravenous steroids are administered. Thrombocytopenia often arises as part of the clinical picture.

63. TTFTF
Aprotinin inhibits proteolytic enzymes, e.g. plasmin (low dose), kallikrein (high dose) and trypsin. It also causes reduced platelet aggregation and has been used in the treatment of pancreatitis although its use is doubtful. KIU stands for kallikrein inactivator units.

64. TFTTT
In an exponential process the rate of change of a quantity at any time is proportional to the quantity at that time. After one half-life the quantity of the substance will have fallen by half. Therefore, after two half-lives the quantity will have fallen by three-quarters. The time constant is the time a process would take to complete if it continued at its initial rate. As the time constant of expiration is equal to the product of lung compliance and lung resistance, high airway resistance requires the period of expiration of a ventilator to be increased. The electrical resistance of a thermistor decreases exponentially as temperature increases.

65. FFFFF
The haematocrit of packed cells is 0.6–0.7. At 22°C platelets have a shelf life of 3–5 days. Using filters leads to platelet fragmentation. Supplies of platelets contain a few red cells and should therefore be ABO-compatible. Cryoprecipitate is rich in fibrinogen.

66. Regarding urinary calculi
  A. Seventy per cent of all calculi are urate calculi
  B. Most calculi develop in the bladder rather than in the upper urinary tract
  C. Primary hypoparathyroidism is a cause of calcium stones
  D. Sarcoidosis causes calcium stones
  E. Calcium stones can occur in low urine output states

67. Regarding inhaled nitric oxide
  A. Methaemoglobinaemia is produced
  B. Nitric oxide binds to haemoglobin as avidly as carbon monoxide
  C. Nitrogen dioxide levels should be monitored
  D. In the treatment of ARDS a suitable inhaled concentration is 5–150 p.p.m.
  E. Nitric oxide shows promise in the treatment of asthmatics

68. Regarding the administration of intravenous fluids
  A. The outer diameter of a 14 standard wire gauge (s.w.g.) cannula is 2.11 mm
  B. A 25 s.w.g. hypodermic needle is blue
  C. In testing the flow rates through different cannulae, distilled water at a constant temperature of 22°C is used
  D. The flow rate through a 14 s.w.g. cannula is 250–360 ml/min
  E. The pH of 4.5% albumin is less than the pH of haemaccel

66. FFFTT
Calcium calculi account for 70% of all urinary calculi. Urate and cystine calculi account for 4% and the remainder are mixed calcium and ammonium phosphate which are due to infection. Seventy-five per cent of urinary calculi patients are male. In the UK most calculi develop in the upper urinary tract. The causes of calcium calculi formation are hypercalcaemia, hypercalciuria, low urine volume, high urine pH, hyperoxaluria, hyperuricosuria and low urinary citrate concentration. The causes of hypercalcaemia are hyperparathyroidism, sarcoidosis, vitamin D ingestion, milk-alkali syndrome, hyperthyroidism and malignant disease.

67. TFTTF
The activity of nitric oxide is terminated by reaction with haemoglobin, which produces methaemoglobin. Nitric oxide binds to haemoglobin more avidly than carbon monoxide. Nitrogen dioxide, an oxidative derivative of nitric oxide, is toxic and levels should be monitored. In ARDS favourable responses occur up to 150 p.p.m. Nitric oxide has not shown promise in the treatment of asthmatics.

68. TFTTF
Colour coding of hypodermic needles is mandatory in the UK. 26 G is brown, 25 G orange, 23 G blue, 22 G black, 21 G green, 20 G yellow and 19 G cream. The flow rate through a 16 s.w.g. canulla is 130–220 ml/min while through an 18 s.w.g. canulla is 75–120 ml/min. All starch and dextran solutions as well as crystalloid solutions, except bicarbonate, are acidic. 4.5% albumin, haemaccel and gelofusin have a pH of 7.4.

69. Concerning anaesthetic breathing systems
   A. To prevent rebreathing when using a Mapleson D breathing system in a spontaneously breathing patient, the fresh gas flow should be 100–150 ml/kg/min
   B. The Humphrey system can perform like a Mapleson A, D or E system depending on the position of a lever situated within the valve block
   C. The Waters' canister is an example of a Mapleson C circuit
   D. When using a vaporizer in circle (VIC) in a ventilated patient, lower than expected concentrations of anaesthetic vapour are delivered to the patient
   E. The taper size of breathing system connections to tracheal tubes is 13 mm

70. When using a nerve stimulator in regional anaesthesia
   A. The anode should be attached to the regional block needle
   B. Insulated needles increase the accuracy
   C. The voltage should be constant
   D. A long stimulation pulse is optimal
   E. Injection should not take place when 0.1 mA stimulates muscle twitching

71. Peritoneal dialysis
   A. Should be used with caution in patients with pulmonary disease
   B. The most common complication is catheter misplacement
   C. Infection may manifest as hypoalbuminaemia
   D. Intravenous broad-spectrum antibiotics are the first line of treatment in peritonitis
   E. May not control uraemia in severely catabolic patients

69. FTFFF

The Mapleson D system is inefficient for spontaneous ventilation as exhaled gas passes into the reservoir bag and is rebreathed. To prevent this, high fresh gas flow rates are required, e.g. 150–250 ml/kg/min, compared with 70 ml/kg/min when using a Mapleson A system. The Waters' canister is a cylindrical drum, which contains soda lime through which patients breathe. When using a vaporizer outside the circle (VOC), the vapour in the circle can be diluted by exhaled gas. The taper size of breathing system connections to tracheal tubes is 15 mm.

70. FTFFT

The cathode should be attached to the regional block needle. To ensure a constant current against tissues with varying resistances the voltage must be variable. A lengthened stimulation pulse reduces accuracy as it reduces the ratio of current required to stimulate the nerve when the needle is 1 cm away, compared with when it is on the nerve. Muscle twitching at 0.1 mA implies intraneuronal needle placement.

71. TFTFT

Due to limitation of diaphragmatic excursion, peritoneal dialysis (PD) should be used with caution in patients with pulmonary disease. The most common complication of PD is infection. Peritonitis leads to increased peritoneal permeability resulting in protein loss. Broad-spectrum antibiotics should be added to the dialysate in the first instance. PD may not control uraemia in severely catabolic patients.

72. **The clinical features and systemic complications of ulcerative colitis include**
    A.   Erythema marginatum
    B.   Ankylosing spondylitis
    C.   Chronic active hepatitis
    D.   Drug-induced fibrosing alveolitis
    E.   Arterial thrombosis

73. **The following statements about parenteral nutrition are true**
    A.   The central route is mandatory
    B.   Amino acids should be administered as D and L forms in equal amounts
    C.   Lipid solutions are iso-osmolar
    D.   5 g of protein will release 1 g of nitrogen
    E.   Linoleic acid is an essential fatty acid

74. **Concerning the measurement of oxygen in the blood**
    A.   Regarding oximetry, 750 nm and 650 nm are the two isobestic points for oxygenated and deoxygenated haemoglobin
    B.   The presence of methaemoglobin leads to a falsely low oxygen saturation reading
    C.   The Clark electrode has a lead anode and platinum cathode and requires a battery to function
    D.   Halothane causes falsely high readings of PO_2 when measured by the Clark electrode
    E.   Hüfner's constant = 1.34 ml in vivo

72. FTTT

Ulcerative colitis is a systemic disease. It affects the gut (diarrhoea, bleeding, tenesmus), constitution (weight loss, malaise, growth retardation), skin (erythema nodosum – marginatum occurs in rheumatic fever!, pyoderma gangenosum), eyes (episcleritis, uveitis), mouth (ulcers), joints (asymmetrical large joint arthropathy, sacro-ileitis, ankylosing spondylitis), liver (fatty liver, chronic active hepatitis, amyloid), biliary system (cholangitis, bile duct carcinoma), lung (sulphasalazine-induced fibrosing alveolitis), kidney (stones, amyloid) and blood (arterial and venous thrombosis). Remember in all questions (both short-answer questions and vivas) that diseases with systemic involvement require answers that reflect the widespread nature of the disease – answers relating only to the gut, with mention of bleeding and electrolytes, are inadequate!

73. FFTFT

Parenteral nutrition may be given both centrally and peripherally. The body can only utilize D-amino acids. Lipid solutions employed in parenteral nutrition are iso-osmolar. 1 g of protein liberates 6.25 g of nitrogen. Linoleic acid is an essential fatty acid.

74. FTFTT

The isobestic points for oxygenated and deoxygenated haemoglobin are 590 and 805 nm. Methaemoglobin is counted as deoxygenated haemoglobin, so that the saturation reading is falsely low. A falsely high saturation is read in the presence of carboxyhaemoglobin, which is counted as oxygenated haemoglobin. The Clark electrode has a silver/silver chloride anode, a platinum cathode and a battery, whereas the fuel cell has a lead anode, a gold cathode and generates its own potential. Hüfner's constant is the volume of oxygen carried by 1 g of haemoglobin. It is equal to 1.34 ml in vivo and 1.39 ml in vitro.

75. Activated clotting time (ACT) is prolonged by
  A. Hypothermia
  B. Dehydration
  C. Antithrombin III deficiency
  D. Hypofibrinogenaemia
  E. Cardioplegic solutions

76. Renal transplantation
  A. Suxamethonium is absolutely contraindicated in the recipient
  B. Maximal donor kidney ischaemic time is 24 h
  C. The donor kidney is placed intra-abdominally in children
  D. Cyclosporin usually causes hypotension after prolonged use
  E. Azathioprine inhibits macrophage production of IL-2

77. Alfentanil
  A. Has a pKa of 8.0
  B. Has a larger volume of distribution than fentanyl
  C. Is more highly protein-bound than fentanyl
  D. Is more lipid-soluble than fentanyl
  E. Is metabolized by the liver

78. The clinical course of human immunodeficiency virus (HIV) infection includes
  A. Seroconversion occurring 3–12 months after exposure to HIV
  B. Fifteen per cent of people experience a glandular fever-like illness at the time of seroconversion
  C. Persistent generalized lymphadenopathy which is usually asymmetrical
  D. Persistent generalized lymphadenopathy which affects the inguinal nodes most commonly
  E. A protozoal opportunistic infection from *Pneumocystis carinii*

75. TFFTT
The normal ACT is 105–167 s. ACT is prolonged by heparin, haemodilution, platelet dysfunction and other coagulopathies, as well as the factors mentioned in the question. Antithrombin III deficiency leads to heparin resistance. An ACT value of >400 s is generally accepted as safe for cardiopulmonary bypass and this usually requires 300 units (3 mg) of heparin per kilogram body weight.

76. FFTFF
Provided the recipient has been dialysed and plasma potassium is not elevated suxamethonium is not contraindicated. The maximum ischaemic time of the donor kidney is 48–72 h. Children are often the recipient of adult kidneys which are most appropriately placed intra-abdominally. Cyclosporin almost invariably causes hypertension with prolonged use. Azathioprine inhibits B and T lymphocyte proliferation.

77. FFTFT
Alfentanil has a pKa of 6.4. It has a smaller volume of distribution than fentanyl (0.4–1.0 and 3–5 l/kg respectively). Alfentanil is 92% protein-bound while fentanyl is 84% protein-bound. It is less lipid-soluble than fentanyl.

78. FFFFF
Seroconversion occurs 3–12 weeks after exposure. 50–80% of people experience glandular fever-like symptoms. Persistent generalized lymphadenopathy is usually symmetrical and most commonly affects the cervical, submandibular and axillary nodes. *P. carinii* was originally classified as a protozoon but has been reclassified as a fungus. The classification of HIV infection as defined by Centers for Disease Control in the USA is: group I (acute infection), group II (asymptomatic infection), group III (persistent generalized lymphadenopathy) and group IV (other manifestations: constitutional, neurological, secondary infections, secondary cancers, other conditions).

79. Conn's syndrome
A. Is rarely caused by a solitary adrenal adenoma (about 15% of cases)
B. Is rarely caused by bilateral hyperplasia of the adrenal glomerulosa cells (about 15% of cases)
C. Is characterized by hypertension and hyperkalaemia
D. Is confirmed by high plasma aldosterone and high plasma renin levels
E. Surgery is recommended for an adenoma but this does not cure the hypertension

80. Cardiac contusions
A. Are often asymptomatic
B. Are associated with aortic valve dysfunction in the young and mitral valve dysfunction in the elderly
C. Delayed cardiac rupture may occur
D. Ventricular aneurysm is a recognized complication
E. Increase in serum creatinine kinase is the most common presentation

81. Concerning the management of hypothermia
A. Pulmonary artery catheters are useful in complex cases
B. When correcting blood gases to hypothermic body temperature the patients are hypercarbic
C. Extracorporeal circulation may be used for rewarming
D. Sodium bicarbonate therapy may be useful
E. Antibiotics should be started prophylactically

79. FTFFF
Primary aldosteronism is relatively uncommon and results from excess production of aldosterone by the zona glomerulosa of the adrenal gland. The causes are a solitary adrenal adenoma (85%) and bilateral hyperplasia (15%). Hyperaldosteronism causes hypertension as a result of salt and water retention. Hypokalaemia classically occurs – it must be remembered before everyone starts diagnosing it in hypertensive patients that the most common cause of hypokalaemia in hypertensive patients is diuretic therapy. A low plasma renin occurs and normally removal of the adenoma will cure the hypertension.

80. TTTTF
Cardiac contusions are often asymptomatic. Compression of the heart in diastole can result in valvular damage. The aortic valve is commonly affected in the young while the mitral valve is more commonly affected in the elderly. Healing is by scarring, which can lead to delayed rupture and ventricular aneurysm formation. ECG abnormalities are the most common presentation.

81. FFTTF
Pulmonary artery catheters should be avoided in cases of hypothermia because of the risk of precipitating ventricular fibrillation. The correction of P_aCO_2 to hypothermic body temperature may result in normocarbia, hypo- or hypercarbia. Extracorporeal circulation has been used to facilitate rewarming. Metabolic acidosis may require treatment with sodium bicarbonate. Antibiotics should only be employed in the presence of established infection.

82. Regarding cardiomyopathy
   A. Hypertrophic obstructive cardiomyopathy (HOCM) is usually caused by alcohol abuse
   B. Digoxin is the treatment of choice in HOCM
   C. Epidural anaesthesia is beneficial in patients with HOCM
   D. Restrictive cardiomyopathy is a side effect of prolonged amiodarone administration
   E. β-blockers are used in the treatment of HOCM

83. The following statements regarding physics are true
   A. Dalton's law relates to the partial pressure of individual gases in a mixture of gases
   B. Charles' law relates the pressure exerted by a constant volume of gas to its temperature
   C. Henry's law states that the rate of diffusion of a substance across a unit area is proportional to the concentration gradient
   D. The Ostwald solubility coefficient is corrected to standard temperature and pressure
   E. The boiling point of oxygen is $-183°C$

82. FFFFT

HOCM is a familial disorder causing hypertrophy of the upper interventricular septum, resulting in left ventricular outflow obstruction. Alcohol, as well as anti-mitotic drugs and sarcoidosis, causes dilated cardiomyopathy, while restrictive cardiomyopathy is caused by fibrosis or infiltration. Digoxin, diuretics, vasodilators and anticoagulants are used in the treatment of dilated cardiomyopathy. Digoxin increases the force of ventricular contraction, thus increasing the degree of outflow obstruction, and is contraindicated in the treatment of HOCM. The converse is true for β-blockers. Peripheral vasodilatation, including epidurals, should be avoided in patients with HOCM. Long-term amiodarone administration causes corneal microdeposits, photosensitivity, peripheral neuropathy, hypo- or hyperthyroidism, hepatitis and pulmonary fibrosis.

83. TFFFT

Dalton's law of partial pressures states that in a mixture of gases the pressure exerted by each gas is equal to the pressure it would exert if it alone occupied the space. Charles' law states that the volume of a given mass of gas at constant pressure varies proportionally with its temperature. The third perfect gas law relates the pressure exerted by a constant volume of gas to its temperature, while Boyle's law states that at constant temperature the volume of a given mass of gas varies inversely with its pressure. Henry's law states that at a particular temperature the amount of a given gas dissolved in a given liquid is directly proportional to the partial pressure of the gas in equilibrium with the liquid. Fick's law states that the rate of diffusion of a substance across a unit area is proportional to the concentration gradient. The Ostwald solubility coefficient is the volume of gas that dissolves in one unit volume of the liquid at the temperature concerned.

84. The malignant neuroleptic syndrome
  A. Is a centrally mediated condition
  B. Is precipitated by MAOI administration
  C. Extrapyramidal signs are not a feature
  D. Onset is rapid
  E. Dantrolene is not useful

85. The neonate with tracheo-oesophageal fistula
  A. The most common abnormality is proximal oesophageal atresia with a fistula connecting the distal trachea and distal oesophagus
  B. The most common site of the fistula is just proximal to the carina
  C. Anal atresia is associated
  D. Fifty per cent of neonates with tracheo-oesophageal fistula are pre-term
  E. Diagnosis is by placement of contrast dye into the proximal oesophagus

86. Signs of infective endocarditis include
  A. Janeway lesions on the hand
  B. Osler's nodes
  C. Clubbing
  D. Nail bed splinter haemorrhages
  E. Splenomegaly

84. TTFFF

The malignant neuroleptic syndrome is a centrally mediated condition secondary to chronic administration of psychotropic drugs, including MAOIs. Extrapyramidal signs are a feature. Malignant neuroleptic syndrome has a gradual onset over weeks to months. Dantrolene is useful in lowering muscle production of heat and hence body temperature.

85. TTTFF

The most common form of this condition is a combination of proximal oesophageal atresia with a fistula connecting the distal oesophagus to the distal trachea, with the fistula entering just above the carina. Thirty per cent of cases are pre-term. Due to the risk of aspiration, radiocontrast dyes are not used to aid diagnosis.

86. TTTTT

Infective endocarditis occurs when the valves or endocardium become infected with organisms, including *Streptococcus viridans*, *Staphylococci aureus* and epidermidis. It can be acute or chronic. Clinical features result from cardiac signs, systemic embolization and immune complex deposition. The immune complex deposits are responsible for the vasculitis: small skin and mucosal haemorrhages, Roth spots (retinal haemorrhages), splinter haemorrhages, red macules on the hand (Janeway complexes) and subcutaneous swellings on the pads of the fingers (Osler's nodes). You must know antibiotic regimens in order to prevent infective endocarditis in patients with peri-operative valve disease.

87. Regarding bundle branch block
  A.   QRS duration is greater than 0.2 s
  B.   Left anterior hemiblock results in left axis deviation
       $>60°$
  C.   Patients with right bundle branch block and left anterior
       hemiblock require pre-operative cardiac pacing
  D.   Right bundle branch block and left posterior hemiblock
       cause left axis deviation $>60°$
  E.   A large S wave in lead I of the ECG is found in patients
       with right bundle branch block

88. Anaphylactic shock
  A.   Anaphylaxis due to neuromuscular blockers occurs
       equally in both males and females
  B.   The majority of anaphylactic reactions to
       neuromuscular blockers occur in the absence of a
       history of prior exposure
  C.   IgE receptors are found on mast cells, basophils and
       eosinophils
  D.   Serum tryptase samples may be taken at post-mortem
  E.   Cardiac output is profoundly depressed

**89. Investigation of the patient with sickle-cell anaemia (SCA)
includes**
  A.   An anaemia of 6–8 g/dl and an elevated reticulocyte
       count of 10–20%
  B.   A peripheral blood film showing sickle cells and target
       cells
  C.   Electrophoresis characterized by migration of a single
       band between HbA2 and HbA
  D.   The 'sickledex' screening test is based on the relative
       insolubility of deoxygenated HbS in solutions of high
       molarity
  E.   Haemoglobin electrophoresis is sometimes necessary to
       confirm SCA

87. FTFFT
In bundle branch block the QRS complex of the ECG must be >0.12 s. Left anterior hemiblock causes left axis deviation >60°, while left posterior hemiblock causes right axis deviation >120°. Bifascicular block involving the right bundle and left anterior fascicle results in an ECG with right bundle branch block and left axis deviation. Right bundle branch block and right axis deviation occur in right bundle branch and left posterior fascicular block. Temporary pacing may be required in patients with bundle branch block associated with a history of syncope or a prolonged PR interval which may progress to complete heart block.

88. FTFTF
Anaphylaxis due to neuromuscular blockers has a male:female incidence ratio of 1:4. More than 50% of anaphylactic reactions to neuromuscular blockers occur in the absence of a history of prior exposure. IgE receptors are not located on eosinophils. Usually cardiac output is not profoundly depressed. Myocardial depression by cytokines is opposed by endogenous adrenaline release.

89. TTTTF
A haemoglobin electrophoresis is always required to confirm sickle-cell disease. In electrophoresis the migration of the single band (HbS) between HbA2 and HbA is at least 70%. The other haematological findings are described in the question. Sickle cells appear irregular and elongated in a peripheral blood film. Target cells and nucleated red cells are often seen as well and they indicate functional hyposplenism, which is often present in patients with sickle-cell disease.

90. The following statements about myxoedema coma are true
 A.   TSH may be low
 B.   TSH may be high
 C.   Seizures may be part of the clinical picture
 D.   Hypernatraemia is a feature
 E.   The mortality rate is 20%

90. TTTFF

Myxoedema coma may result from primary hypothyroidism, giving a high TSH or, more rarely, a hypothalamic or pituitary lesion giving a low TSH. Hyponatraemia occurs and is usually mild; however, when severe, it causes fitting. Mortality is of the order of 50%.

Paper 3

1. **The following refer to carcinoid syndrome**
   A. Somatostatin reduces the release of serotonin from carcinoid tumours
   B. Intra-operative hypotension resistant to fluid replacement should be treated with ephedrine rather than methoxamine
   C. 100 µg subcutaneous octreotide is useful as a premedicant in patients with carcinoid syndrome
   D. Kallikrein is a protease enzyme responsible for the production of bradykinin
   E. Ketanserin is used in patients with carcinoid syndrome to treat flushing associated with bradykinin release

2. **Concerning carbon dioxide**
   A. The partial pressure of carbon dioxide in venous blood is 6.1 kPa
   B. Carbon dioxide has a molecular weight of 44
   C. Carbon dioxide has a critical temperature of $-31°C$
   D. Carbon dioxide is supplied in cylinders at a pressure of 50 bar at room temperature
   E. Deoxygenated haemoglobin carries more carbon dioxide than oxygenated haemoglobin because it has an increased ability to form carbamino groups

3. **Regarding the physiology of vomiting**
   A. The chemoreceptor trigger zone (CTZ) lies within the blood–brain barrier in the floor of the IVth ventricle
   B. $5\text{-}HT_3$, dopamine (D_2), acetylcholine (M_3) and histamine (H_1) receptors are found in the CTZ
   C. Opioids stimulate µ receptors in the CTZ, causing nausea
   D. Hyperkalaemia is a potent stimulus of chemoreceptors located adjacent to the CTZ
   E. The vomiting centre lies within the blood–brain barrier

1. **TFTTF**
   Sympathomimetic drugs can trigger the release of carcinoid peptides from carcinoid tumours and should not be used in the treatment of intra-operative hypotension in these patients. Initial management includes intravenous fluid therapy and asking the surgeon to stop manipulating the tumour. Further treatment includes octreotide, vasopressin and aprotinin. Flushing is due to both histamine and bradykinin release. Antihistamines treat flushing associated with histamine release, while aprotinin, a kallikrein inhibitor, prevents bradykinin production. Ketanserin blocks the effects of serotonin on the 5-HT_2 receptor and has α-adrenergic antagonist activity.

2. **TTFFT**
   The critical temperature of carbon dioxide is +31°C so that at room temperature it is a vapour. Carbon dioxide is supplied in grey cylinders with a pressure of 50 bar at 15°C and 57 bar at room temperature. Carbon dioxide in venous red blood cells is converted to carbonic acid, which dissociates into bicarbonate and hydrogen ions. Bicarbonate is exchanged for chloride ions in the plasma while hydrogen ions are buffered by haemoglobin. Deoxygenated haemoglobin has a greater ability at buffering hydrogen ions and forming carbamino groups than oxygenated haemoglobin (Haldane effect).

3. **FTFFT**
   The CTZ lies in the area postrema, outside the blood–brain barrier, unlike the vomiting centre which it stimulates and which is located in the dorsolateral reticular formation of the brainstem within the blood–brain barrier. Opioids may cause release of dopamine within the CTZ, leading to stimulation of D_2 receptors and emesis. Hyperkalaemia has no effect on vomiting.

4. Tramadol
   A.   Is presented as a racemic mixture
   B.   Has half the analgesic potency of pethidine
   C.   Inhibits the release of serotonin
   D.   Should be used with caution in patients taking MAOIs
   E.   Is a weak μ-receptor agonist

5. In renal failure
   A.   Increased renin secretion occurs which causes hypertension
   B.   Decreased erythropoietin secretion occurs which causes anaemia
   C.   Decreased hydroxylation of vitamin D_2 to form vitamin D_3 occurs which causes renal osteodystrophy
   D.   Impaired sodium and water balance occurs which causes hypovolaemia due to salt wasting
   E.   Decreased plasma calcium and phosphate contributes to the renal osteodystrophy

6. Hypercalcaemia of malignancy occurs in
   A.   Cerebral astrocytoma
   B.   Primary malignant melanoma
   C.   Uterine carcinoma
   D.   Ovarian carcinoma
   E.   Carcinoma of the large bowel

4. TFFFT
Tramadol has the same analgesic potency as pethidine. A proportion of its analgesic activity is mediated by enhanced release of serotonin, resulting in spinal inhibition of nociception. Because of this enhancement of monoaminergic transmission it is contraindicated in patients receiving MAOIs.

5. FTTTT
The pathophysiology of renal failure can be basically divided into two parts: disturbed endocrine regulation and failed excretory regulation. The endocrine regulation is decreased erythropoietin and renin secretion and decreased hydroxylation of vitamin D_2 to D_3. This results in anaemia, hypertension and renal osteodystrophy. The failed excretory regulation is more complex and is six-fold in nature: impaired sodium and water balance, hyperkalaemia, increased hydrogen ions, increased urea, decreased plasma calcium and phosphate, and increased other nitrogenous waste products (middle molecules). These respectively cause cardiac failure, arrhythmias, acidosis, nausea and vomiting, renal osteodystrophy, and the uraemic syndrome.

6. FFFTF
Hypercalcaemia of malignancy occurs in 5% of patients with malignancy in hospitals and there are five malignancies that it is commonly associated with. These are squamous cell carcinoma of the lung, adenocarcinoma of the breast, renal carcinoma, ovarian carcinoma and haematogenous tumours (especially multiple myeloma). Biochemical findings include reduced serum phosphate, reduced parathormone: while the alkaline phosphatase and serum creatinine may be elevated, especially if dehydration is present.

7. **The adult trachea**
   A. Is 12 cm long
   B. Commences opposite C6
   C. The thyroid isthmus covers rings 3–6
   D. The brachiocephalic artery is a close anterior relation
   E. The azygous vein runs on the left side

8. **The cadaveric organ donor**
   A. Is likely to be hyponatraemic
   B. Corneas must be removed within the first 12 h
   C. Malignant disease precludes organ donation
   D. Atropine will produce a brisk tachycardia
   E. Hypoglycaemia is common due to reduced cortisol levels

9. **Concerning drug handling in burns patients**
   A. Renal clearance of gentamicin increases
   B. The peak plasma concentration of vancomycin is reduced
   C. The elimination half-life of cimetidine is reduced
   D. The elimination half-life of ranitidine is unchanged
   E. The volume of distribution of ranitidine increases

10. **Concerning the flow of gases**
    A. Turbulent flow will occur at a higher gas velocity if a patient is breathing air rather than a 60% N_2O:40% O_2 gas mixture
    B. Turbulent flow occurs at lower gas flow rates the narrower the endotracheal tube
    C. During the respiratory cycle, peak inspiratory flow rate in an adult is approximately 100 l/min
    D. In a gas mixture of 60% N_2O:40% O_2, turbulent flow occurs at a flow rate of 22 l/min in anaesthetic tubing with an internal diameter of 22 mm
    E. For the same gas flow rate, warm gases are more prone to turbulence than cooler gases

7. FTFTF

The adult trachea is 15 cm long and commences opposite C6. The thyroid isthmus overlies rings 2–4. The brachiocephalic artery is closely related anteriorly to the trachea. The azygous vein lies on the right side of the trachea.

8. FFFFF

Due to reduced levels of ADH, diabetes insipidus is very common, causing hypernatraemia. The corneas must be removed within the first 24 h. Primary brain tumours do not exclude organ donation. Atropine is not effective, as the vagus nerve is no longer functioning. Although cortisol levels drop, hyperglycaemia is the usual feature of brainstem death.

9. TTTTT

Gentamicin has a lower peak plasma level in burns patients; this is due to an increase in clearance without changes in volume of distribution. Vancomycin levels are also lower in burns patients due to an increased glomerular filtration rate. Cimetidine has a reduced elimination half-life due to an increased clearance. The elimination half-life of ranitidine is unchanged as although clearance increases its volume of distribution also increases.

10. FTFTF

The likelihood of turbulent flow (Reynold's number) is proportional to the diameter of the tube in which the gas flows and the linear velocity and density of the gas, and is inversely proportional to its viscosity. A 60% N_2O:40% O_2 gas mixture is less dense than air so that flow will become turbulent at a higher gas velocity. Similarly, a warm gas is less dense than a cool gas so that at a given flow rate turbulent flow will be less likely. For a standard anaesthetic mixture, the critical flow rate (l/min) equals the diameter of the tube (mm) in which it flows. The peak flow rate in the respiratory cycle is about 50 l/min.

11. **Concerning intravenous fluids**
    A. Sodium chloride 0.9% has a pH of 7.0
    B. Dextrose 5% has a pH of 4.5
    C. Hartmann's solution has a pH of 7.4
    D. Sodium chloride 0.9% is mildly hypotonic
    E. The average molecular weight of Hetastarch is 450 000

12. **Factors that point to an increased likelihood of post-operative ventilation in patients with myasthenia gravis include**
    A. Duration of myasthenia gravis
    B. History of chronic respiratory disease
    C. Dose of pyridostigmine pre-operatively
    D. Vital capacity <2.9 l
    E. Patient age

13. **The clinical features of sickle-cell anaemia include**
    A. Acute respiratory distress syndrome
    B. Convulsions
    C. Cardiomegaly
    D. Paraplegia
    E. *Salmonella* infections

14. **Fat embolus syndrome**
    A. Is associated with pancreatitis
    B. A patent foramen ovale has been implicated in its development
    C. Fifty per cent of all major trauma patients at post-mortem have evidence of fat embolus
    D. Fat globules may be detected in the urine
    E. Is associated with an increased P_aCO_2

11. FTFFT

All these fluids are found in theatre and make very interesting reading during hysterectomies! Sodium chloride 0.9% has a pH of 6.0. Five per cent dextrose has a pH of 4.5 and Hartmann's solution has a pH of 6.5. Sodium chloride 0.9% is isotonic. The average molecular weight of Hetastarch is 450 000.

12. TTTTF

In predicting the likelihood of post-operative ventilation, four risk factors have been identified. The duration of myasthenia gravis has the greatest predictive value. A history of chronic respiratory disease other than respiratory dysfunction secondary to myasthenia gravis. A daily dose of pyridostigmine >750 mg and a vital capacity below 2.9 l are predictive.

13. TTTFT

Most people with sickle-cell anaemia are well except for the acute painful infarct episodes or when an acute haemolytic or aplastic crisis occurs. Parvovirus infections often cause these complications. Other features that occur include acute respiratory distress syndrome, cardiac hypertrophy, infections, leg ulcers, progressive glomerular sclerosis, priapism, hemiplegia and convulsions. Infections caused by *Salmonella*, *Pneumococcus*, and *Haemophilus influenzae* are common.

14. TTFTF

Fat embolus syndrome has been described in association with acute pancreatitis. Mental insufficiency has two postulated aetiologies: firstly hypoxaemia and secondly the passage of paradoxical emboli through a patent foramen ovale. Ninety per cent is the quoted incidence of fat emboli at post-mortem following major trauma. Fat globules may be detected in the urine. Respiratory insufficiency causes an increased respiratory rate with consequent decrease in P_aCO_2.

15. Fulminant hepatic failure
A. May occur in the absence of encephalopathy
B. Prophylactic FFP is beneficial
C. Alcohol abuse is the most common world-wide cause
D. The underlying aetiology has a minor influence on the prognosis
E. May necessitate the use of intracranial pressure monitoring

16. The adult respiratory distress syndrome
A. Mortality rate is of the order of 40%
B. Mortality rate is independent of precipitating cause
C. On bronchioalveolar lavage protein content is equal to that of cardiogenic pulmonary oedema
D. There are areas of both high and low V/Q mismatch
E. FRC remains unchanged

17. Tumour necrosis factor α
A. Binds to renal, lung and liver receptors
B. Levels are raised in both alcoholic hepatitis and congestive cardiac failure
C. Is released from natural killer cells
D. Is a myocardial depressant
E. Increases thromboxane A_2 formation

15. **FFFFT**

    Fulminant hepatic failure (FHF) by definition includes encephalopathy occurring within the first 8 weeks of the onset of symptoms. FHF is associated with a complex array of clotting abnormalities; however, the administration of prophylactic FFP to patients who are not bleeding is not associated with improved outcome. The most common cause world-wide is viral in aetiology. Underlying aetiology has a major influence on outcome. Intracranial pressure monitoring has been used in the management of cerebral oedema in FHF.

16. **FFFTF**

    The mortality in adult respiratory distress syndrome (ARDS) is >50% and is highly dependent on the precipitating cause. The protein content of the exudate is higher in ARDS than in cardiogenic pulmonary oedema. ARDS is associated with areas of both high and low V/Q mismatch and a reduced FRC.

17. **TTTTT**

    Tumour necrosis factor α binds preferentially to renal, liver and lung receptors. Levels are raised in response to endotoxin and various other conditions, including congestive cardiac failure and alcoholic hepatitis. Although predominantly released from macrophages it is also released from natural killer cells. Tumour necrosis factor α is a myocardial depressant. By increasing the metabolism of arachidonic acid it increases the formation of thromboxane A_2.

18. Fibrinolysis is inhibited by
    A.   Tranexamic acid
    B.   Aprotinin
    C.   Aspirin
    D.   Aminocaproic acid
    E.   Catecholamines

19. Examples of double lumen tubes
    A.   The White tube is a left-sided tube
    B.   The Bryce–Smith tube has a carinal hook
    C.   The Carlens tube was invented primarily for lung isolation during surgery
    D.   The Carlens tube does not have a carinal hook
    E.   The Robertshaw tube has the largest lumina

20. Vaporizers
    A.   The TEC 3 has a temperature-compensation device at the entrance to the vaporization chamber
    B.   The OMV is temperature-compensated
    C.   The OMV has a copper heat sink
    D.   The Goldman vaporizer may be used with halothane
    E.   The EMO may be used with a variety of volatile agents

21. The clinical signs and features of Cushing's syndrome include
    A.   Depression
    B.   Hypomania
    C.   Distal myopathy
    D.   Associated Paget's disease
    E.   Hypokalaemic hypertension

18. TTFTF

Low-dose aprotinin inhibits plasmin, causing reduced fibrinolysis. In contrast, at medium dose it prevents platelet aggregation. Aspirin has no effect on fibrinolysis but does inhibit platelet cyclo-oxygenase, causing reduced platelet aggregation. Aminocaproic acid and tranexamic acid inhibit plasminogen activation to plasmin and thus reduce fibrinolysis. Catecholamines increase fibrinolysis.

19. FFFFT

The White tube is a right-sided tube. The Bryce–Smith tube does not have a carinal hook. The Carlens tube was invented primarily for differential bronchospirometry and is a left-sided tube with a carinal hook. The Robertshaw tube has the largest lumina of the double-lumen tubes.

20. FFFTF

The TEC 3 vaporizer has a bimetallic strip at the entrance to the bypass chamber. The OMV is not temperature-compensated but it does have a water heat sink. The Goldman vaporizer is used with potent agents such as halothane. The EMO vaporizer may only be used with ether.

21. TTFFT

In Cushing's syndrome 90% of patients show psychiatric features which range from depression (common) to psychotic mania (rare). They have a proximal myopathy and develop osteoporosis. Patients have thin skin, hirsutism, acne, striae and bruise easily. Hyperglycaemia is common and the musculoskeletal signs include a moon face, hump, truncal obesity and thin limbs.

22. Consequences of permissive hypercapnia include
  A.   Raised pulmonary artery occlusion pressure
  B.   Decreased shunt fraction
  C.   Reduced peak airway pressure
  D.   Hypokalaemia
  E.   Raised intracranial pressure

23. Regarding brachial plexus block
  A.   The ulnar nerve is derived from the medial cord of the brachial plexus
  B.   Scalenus medius inserts into the scalene tubercle of the first rib
  C.   The radial nerve only contains contributions from the C5–C7 nerve roots
  D.   The lateral cutaneous nerve of the forearm is a continuation of the musculocutaneous nerve
  E.   Ptosis, enophthalmos and mydriasis are complications of brachial plexus block

24. The following are associated with pregnancy
  A.   A rise in systemic vascular resistance
  B.   A 20% increase in dead space by term
  C.   A mild respiratory acidosis by the third trimester
  D.   A 10–15% increase in cardiac output by term
  E.   An increased sensitivity to vasopressors

22. TFTFT

Pulmonary artery occlusion pressure rises secondary to increased cardiac output and pulmonary vasoconstriction mediated by concomitant acidosis. Shunt fraction increases due to alveolar derecruitment. Reduced peak airway pressure is a consequence of reduced tidal volume. Hyperkalaemia results due to renal conservation of potassium ions in an attempt to correct acidosis. Increased P_aCO_2 leads to increased cerebral blood flow and consequent raised intracranial pressure.

23. TFFTF

Scalenus anterior inserts into the scalene tubercle of the first rib while scalenus medius inserts into the first rib behind the groove for the subclavian artery. The roots of the brachial plexus lie in the interscalene groove. The radial nerve is the terminal branch of the posterior cord of the brachial plexus and contains nerve fibres from the C5–T1 nerve roots. The musculocutaneous nerve is derived from the lateral cord of the brachial plexus. Horner's syndrome, a complication of brachial plexus and stellate ganglion block, includes ptosis, enophthalmos, lack of sweating, nasal stuffiness and miosis and is due to block of the sympathetic innervation.

24. FFFFF

Pulmonary and systemic vascular resistance fall by about 21% and 34% respectively during pregnancy. In general, pregnant women are less responsive to vasopressors and chronotropes. Dead space is unaltered during pregnancy although both tidal volume (50%) and respiratory rate (15%) increase by term. These are responsible for a 70% increase in alveolar ventilation, a fall in arterial PCO_2 and a mild respiratory alkalosis. Cardiac output increases by as much as 50% by term, primarily due to a 50% increase in stroke volume.

25. Regarding blood transfusion
A. Three per cent of the UK population are blood group B
B. SAG-M blood contains saline, adenine, glutamine and mannitol
C. The pore size of screen filters in standard blood-giving sets is 170 μm
D. In stored blood the levels of clotting factors IX and X start to fall after 7 days
E. Platelets stored at 22°C survive for 10 days

26. Retrobulbar block
A. Lowers intraocular pressure
B. The eye should be looking superonasally
C. Obicularis oculi is not blocked
D. Risk of globe perforation is increased in myopic individuals
E. Requires higher volumes of local anaesthetic than peribulbar block

27. Regarding urinary tract infections
A. Sickle-cell disease does not predispose to urinary tract infections
B. Microbiological midstream urine with >10 000 bacterial colonies per millilitre indicates acute infection
C. The commonest causative organism is *Proteus mirabilis*
D. Thirty per cent of *E. coli* are resistant to amoxycillin
E. Bacteriuria in pregnancy must always be treated

25. FFTTF

Forty-two per cent of the UK population are blood group A, 8% group B, 3% group AB and 47% group O. SAG-M blood contains saline 140 mmol/l, adenine 1.5 mmol/l, glucose 50 mmol/l and mannitol 30 mmol/l. Filtration of microaggregates requires filters of 20–40 μm but the use of these filters is controversial. The survival time for platelets stored at 22°C is 3–5 days. This time is greatly reduced in blood stored at 2–6°C.

26. FFTTF

Retrobulbar block does not consistently lower intraocular pressure. Looking superonasally increases the risk of perforation of the globe, as well as injection into the optic nerve or ophthalmic artery. The eye should be in primary gaze. Myopia increases the anteroposterior diameter of the globe, increasing the risk of perforation. Lower volumes are used in retrobulbar block.

27. FFFTT

Polycystic kidney and sickle-cell disease predispose to urinary tract infections. Diabetes may present with a urinary tract infection. Midstream urine must contain >100 000 bacterial colonies/millilitre in active infection. The commonest organism is still *E. coli* (68%). Other causative organisms include *P. mirabilis* (12%), *Staphylococcus epidermidis* (10%), *Streptococcus faecalis* (6%) and *Klebsiella aerogenes* (4%). Acute pyelonephritis develops in 25% of pregnant women if bacteriuria in pregnancy is left untreated and this can increase perinatal mortality in late pregnancy.

28. Cisapride
 A. Is a central, indirectly acting cholinergic drug
 B. Has an oral bioavailability of 20%
 C. Has low protein binding
 D. The bioavailability of ranitidine is increased when given
    with cisapride
 E. Has a half-life of 3 h

29. Regarding solubility
 A. Bunsen's solubility coefficient is independent of
    temperature and pressure while Ostwald's solubility
    coefficient is measured at standard temperature and
    pressure (s.t.p.)
 B. The relationship between the oil/gas partition coefficient
    and the MAC value of volatile anaesthetic agents at
    $37°C$ is a linear one
 C. The blood gas solubility partition coefficient of xenon is
    greater than that of nitrous oxide
 D. Halothane is more soluble than enflurane in rubber
 E. The vapour pressure of a solvent is increased by the
    addition of a solute

30. Concerning altitude
 A. The rotameters of an anaesthetic machine are unaffected
    by altitude
 B. Oxygen saturation of haemoglobin is maintained at
    >90% up to altitudes of 10 000 feet when no
    supplemental oxygen is given
 C. At room temperature, ether will boil at an altitude of
    18 000 feet
 D. When breathing air at 20 000 feet, the FIO_2 value is 0.17
 E. Hypoxia increases pulmonary vascular resistance

28. FFFFF
Pharmacology questions require two things: understanding of pharmacokinetics and learning. This learning just has to be done and knowledge of new drugs is required for the examination. Cisapride is an indirectly acting peripheral cholinergic drug and, as a consequence, is largely devoid of central depressant and antidopaminergic effects. The drug has a bioavailability of 40–50%, is highly protein-bound and has a half-life of 10 h. It reduces the activity of ranitidine.

29. FFFTF
The Bunsen solubility coefficient is the volume of gas measured at s.t.p. dissolved in unit volume of liquid at the stated temperature and pressure. The Ostwald solubility coefficient is the volume of gas that dissolves in a unit volume of liquid at the stated temperature and pressure. Therefore, at $0°C$ the Ostwald solubility coefficient equals the Bunsen solubility coefficient. A linear relationship exists between oil/gas partition coefficient and MAC of volatile anaesthetic agents only when the $\log_{10}$ values of both are plotted against each other. The blood gas coefficients of xenon and nitrous oxide are 0.17 and 0.47 respectively. Raoult's law states that the vapour pressure of a solvent is lowered if a solute is added to it.

30. FTTFT
At altitude the atmospheric pressure is reduced so that the volume of a given gas will increase. It is therefore less dense. As the height of the bobbin in the flow meter is maintained by gas molecules hitting it, the less dense the gas, the greater the flow has to be to keep the bobbin at the same height. Therefore at altitude the flow meters under-read. The saturated vapour pressure of ether (425 mmHg) is greater than the atmospheric pressure at 18 000 feet (325 mmHg) and it will therefore boil. The FIO_2 value of air at any altitude is 21%. However, the PO_2 value will be reduced as altitude increases and atmospheric pressure decreases.

31. **Concerning drugs and cardiopulmonary bypass**
    A. Nitroprusside toxicity is potentially increased
    B. Following bypass, digoxin levels drop
    C. Plasma pancuronium levels alter due to changes in protein binding
    D. Digoxin is adsorbed onto the bypass circuit
    E. At initiation of bypass there is a small drop in plasma fentanyl levels

32. **Phantom limb pain**
    A. Occurs in up to 50% of amputees
    B. Is worsened if pre-amputation pain is present
    C. Pre-amputation epidurals are useful in reducing incidence of phantom pain
    D. Pain remains constant with time
    E. Severity is independent of extent of amputation

33. **Regarding the treatment of thyrotoxicosis**
    A. Propylthiouracil can cause agranulocytosis
    B. Propylthiouracil is often preferred in pregnant patients because it is less teratogenic than carbimazole
    C. Propranolol directly reduces the conversion of T_4 to T_3
    D. Potassium iodide reduces gland vascularity if given 10 days prior to surgery
    E. A transient hypercalcaemia can arise after surgery due to parathyroid gland damage

31. TFFFF
Nitroprusside is non-enzymatically degraded to cyanide in a temperature-independent process. However, the metabolism of cyanide is a temperature-dependent process and therefore may be reduced by hypothermia during cardiopulmonary bypass (CPB). The reduction in plasma pancuronium levels is secondary to haemodilution rather than changes in protein binding, as it is <50% protein-bound. Digoxin is not adsorbed to the CPB circuit. At initiation of CPB there is a rapid, large drop in plasma fentanyl levels secondary to haemodilution and increased volume of distribution.

32. FTTFF
Phantom limb pain occurs in up to 85% of amputees. Pre-amputation epidurals lasting for 72 h have been shown to be useful. Phantom pain gradually recedes over time. The degree of phantom pain is related to the extent of the amputation.

33. FTTTF
Carbimazole is the most commonly used drug – it is a thiourea that inhibits the production and coupling of iodotyrosine and thereby inhibits thyroid hormone production. It only causes two side effects of interest to anaesthetists, namely skin rashes and agranulocytosis. Propranolol is used for tremors and palpitations. A transient hypocalcaemia may occur post surgery following parathyroid damage. Anaesthetic-based questions on the thyroid require complete answers: pre-operative assessment of thyroid status, drugs, atrial fibrillation, exophthalmos and airway problems are important.

34. The following statements regarding physical properties are true
  A. Desflurane is a vapour at room temperature
  B. Raoult's law relates to the lowering of temperature which occurs when a gas expands
  C. One coulomb is the amount of charge passing any point in an electrical circuit in 1 s when a current of 1 A is flowing
  D. Fick's law of diffusion relates the rate of diffusion across a membrane to the cross-sectional area of the membrane
  E. The vapours of isoflurane and enflurane are lighter than air

35. Regarding the human immunodeficiency virus (HIV)
  A. 0.3% of people become infected with HIV following a needle-stick injury from an infected patient
  B. Perinatal transmission from the mother to the child occurs in 95% of cases
  C. Breast feeding carries no risk of HIV transmission to the child
  D. HIV is a DNA retrovirus
  E. The main target for HIV is the T-helper lymphocyte

36. The following statements are true regarding the APACHE II scoring system
  A. Measurement of the physiological variables is performed during the first 12 h after admission
  B. Thirty-four physiological variables are measured
  C. The maximum score is 83
  D. It allows comparison between different ITUs
  E. Blood lactate is one of the physiological variables

34. FFTFF
Raoult's law describes the lowering of vapour pressure of a solvent if a solute is added to it. The Joule–Thomson, or Joule–Kelvin, effect explains the fall in temperature when a gas expands. It is the principle employed by the cryoprobe. Fick's law states that the rate of diffusion of a substance across a membrane is proportional to its concentration gradient, while Graham's law states that the rate of diffusion of a gas is inversely proportional to the square root of its molecular weight. The vapours of isoflurane and enflurane are 7.5 times heavier than air.

35. TFFFT
HIV is transmitted sexually, via blood, and perinatally to the child from the mother. Perinatal transmission occurs in about 16–30% of cases. Breast feeding carries a small but definite risk to the child. HIV is a RNA retrovirus. The virus binds to a glycoprotein on the surface of the T cell (CD4) and then enters the cell causing dysfunction.

36. FFFTF
Measurement of physiological variables is during the first 24 h after admission to ITU. The APACHE II scoring system measures 12 physiological variables. It has a maximum score of 71. The APACHE II scoring system allows comparison between different ITUs. Blood lactate is not a feature of the APACHE II scoring system.

37. Precautions used in theatre to minimize the risks of injury due to electricity
   A.   Micro shock is less likely if normal saline, rather than 5% dextrose, is used in centrally placed catheters
   B.   The theatre floor should have a resistance of 10 000–20 000 ohms between two points 60 cm apart
   C.   Antistatic rubber equipment should have a resistance of at least 100 000 ohms/cm
   D.   Class II electrical equipment must be earthed
   E.   Relative humidity should be <50% to prevent sparks occurring due to static discharge

38. Selective decontamination of the digestive tract
   A.   Maintains the normal aerobic flora
   B.   Antibiotic therapy is given orally and via the nasogastric tube
   C.   Amphotericin B is an intravenous component
   D.   Involves the use of parenteral antibiotics
   E.   Lowers overall mortality

37. **FFTFF**
Micro shock is less likely if non-ion-containing fluids such as 5% dextrose are used in central lines as they do not conduct electricity. To allow static charge to leak away, equipment, flooring and theatre shoes should have a low enough resistance to allow some flow of current to earth while being high enough to prevent electrocution. Black antistatic rubber equipment, which has a yellow identification label, has a resistance of 100 000–10 000 000 ohms/cm while terrazzo flooring should have a resistance of 20 000–5 000 000 ohms between two points 60 cm apart. Class I equipment must be earthed and contain a fuse. Class II equipment must be doubly insulated and no earth is required. With class III equipment no potential greater than 24 V is allowed, making macro shock unlikely. Sparks are more likely in cold dry atmospheres, so the relative humidity should be >50% and the temperature >20°C.

38. **FTFTF**
Selective decontamination of the digestive tract aims to eliminate aerobic gut organisms while preserving the normal anaerobic flora. To prevent infection by fungal organisms enteral amphotericin B is a component of treatment. Intravenous antibiotics are also administered. Selective decontamination of the digestive tract has not been shown to lower overall mortality.

39. Concerning inotropes

  A. Phosphodiesterase inhibitors, e.g. milrinone, increase diastolic compliance, relaxation and filling of the left ventricle
  B. Glucagon is a positive inotrope
  C. Dopamine infusion causes nausea and vomiting by stimulation of D_2 receptors in the vomiting centre
  D. Dopexamine is a potent β_2 agonist
  E. Tachyphylaxis can occur to dobutamine after 72 h administration

40. Recognized strategies for the management of hypoxia during one lung anaesthesia include

  A. Fibre optic bronchoscopy
  B. Application of CPAP to the non-dependent lung
  C. Application of PEEP to the dependent lung
  D. Lowering the tidal volume
  E. Clamping the pulmonary artery

39. TTFTT

The beneficial effects of phosphodiesterase inhibitors on the ventricle, namely better diastolic compliance, filling and relaxation, occur at lower doses than those required to produce inotropy. Glucagon binds to specific receptors on the heart, distinct from β receptors, resulting in an increase in intracellular cAMP, Ca^{2+} influx and positive inotropy. Glucagon causes significant nausea, vomiting and hyperglycaemia and is only used for the emergency treatment of β-antagonist overdose. Peripherally administered dopamine does not cross the blood–brain barrier and so has no effect on the D_2 receptors in the vomiting centre. Dopexamine has a 60 times more potent effect on the β_2 receptor than dopamine. It also has minor β_1 activity, and some activity on both D_1 and D_2 receptors. It is a potent catecholamine re-uptake inhibitor.

40. TTTTT

Malposition of the double lumen tube causing hypoxia may be identified by fibre optic bronchoscopy. The application of CPAP to the non-dependent lung and PEEP to the dependent lung have both been shown to increase oxygenation. Excessive tidal volumes lead to increased dependent lung vascular resistance and hence non-dependent lung blood flow. Refractory hypoxaemia may be managed by clamping the pulmonary artery to the non-dependent lung. This eliminates all shunt flow through the non-dependent lung.

41. The clinical signs and symptoms of lithium toxicity include
  A. Hepatic failure
  B. Coarse tremor
  C. Dry mouth
  D. Convulsions
  E. Sick sinus syndrome

42. Pseudocholinesterase
  A. Suxamethonium is oxidized to form succinic acid
  B. Pseudocholinesterase deficiency is inherited as an autosomal recessive gene
  C. Pseudocholinesterase is inhibited by cyclophosphamide
  D. A dibucaine number of 75–85 is found in people with the normal enzyme
  E. A fluoride number of 60 is found in the normal population

43. Regarding the nerve supply and topical anaesthesia of the nose
  A. The nerve supply to the nose is from the maxillary and zygomatic branches of the trigeminal nerve
  B. The maxillary antrum is supplied by the maxillary division of the trigeminal nerve via the shenopalatine ganglion
  C. The anterior and posterior branches of the nasociliary nerve supply the ethmoid region of the nose
  D. Moffet's solution contains 2 ml 8% cocaine, 2 ml 1% sodium bicarbonate and 1 ml 1:1000 adrenaline
  E. The frontal sinus is supplied by the frontal branch of the maxillary nerve

44. Post-herpetic neuralgia
  A. Is more common in the elderly
  B. Rarely involves the trigeminal nerve
  C. Is frequently unilateral
  D. Allodynia is a feature
  E. TENS is ineffective

41. FTFTF

Lithium is contraindicated in patients with pre-existing renal impairment and the sick sinus syndrome. Side effects in the therapeutic range include nausea, metallic taste, fine tremor, nephrogenic diabetes insipidus, hypothyroidism and weight gain. In the toxic range the side effects are vomiting, diarrhoea, coarse tremor, ataxia, seizures, coma and distal tubular degeneration. Toxicity has a high mortality and is associated with irreversible renal and neurological damage. Blood levels should be monitored every 4 months and the serum level should be 0.5–1.2 mmol/l. In addition, thyroid function should be checked every 6 months.

42. FTTTT

Pseudocholinesterase hydrolyses suxamethonium to succinic acid. Pseudocholinesterase is inhibited by cyclophosphamide, ecothiopate and phenelzine. It is deficient in pregnancy, hepatic failure, hypoproteinaemia, malnutrition and after plasmapheresis. The normal enzyme has a dibucaine number (DN) of 75–85 and a fluoride number (FN) of 60. The atypical enzyme has a DN of 15–25 and an FN of 20. The fluoride-resistant enzyme has a DN of 65–75 but an FN of only 30.

43. FTTTF

The nerve supply to the nose is from the first two (ophthalmic and maxillary) divisions of the trigeminal nerve. The frontal nerve, a branch of the ophthalmic division of the trigeminal nerve, supplies the frontal sinus.

44. TFTTF

Post-herpetic neuralgia occurs almost exclusively above the age of 50. Most often it involves the thoracic dermatomes and the ophthalmic division of the trigeminal nerve. It is frequently unilateral. Allodynia is a feature. TENS has been shown to be a useful treatment.

45. **Signs and symptoms of tricyclic antidepressant overdose include**
    A.   Hallucinations
    B.   Urinary frequency
    C.   Diarrhoea
    D.   Hypertension
    E.   Metabolic alkalosis

46. **Concerning pulmonary artery rupture complicating pulmonary artery catheterization**
    A.   Mortality is up to 60%
    B.   The most common cause is erosion by the catheter tip
    C.   Pulmonary hypertension is a risk factor
    D.   Successful treatments include pulmonary resection
    E.   Hypothermic cardiopulmonary bypass theoretically increases the risk

47. **Regarding anti-arrhythmic drugs**
    A.   Class IV drugs increase the PR interval of the ECG
    B.   Class IV drugs include sotalol and amiodarone
    C.   Adenosine acts on the atrioventricular node by stimulating adenosine receptors
    D.   The therapeutic serum concentration of digoxin is 10–14 ng/l
    E.   Nimodipine is a calcium channel blocker which acts predominantly on cerebral blood vessels

45. TFFFF

Overdose leads to fatalities as a result of the action of these drugs on the heart and central nervous system. The anticholinergic actions lead to dilated pupils, tachycardia, urinary retention, ileus and hallucinations. The central effects cause convulsions and the cardiac problems cause hypotension and arrhythmias. Metabolic acidosis subsequently occurs. These drugs have an 'apparent void of distribution' and blood levels are not indicative of potential clinical problems.

46. FFTTT

Pulmonary artery rupture following pulmonary artery catheterization has a mortality of up to 83%. The most common cause of rupture is secondary to balloon overinflation rather than erosion. Risk factors include pulmonary hypertension. Successful treatment has involved pulmonary resection. During hypothermic cardiopulmonary bypass the catheter tip becomes stiffer and migrates distally, theoretically increasing the risk of rupture.

47. TFTFT

Class IV drugs, e.g. verapamil, nifedipine, nimodipine and diltiazem, block the slow influx of calcium into the sinoatrial node, prolonging the PR interval, and therefore have some use in the treatment of supraventricular arrhythmias. Sotalol has properties of both class II (β-blockers) and class III drugs. Class III drugs, which include amiodarone and bretylium, prolong the duration of the action potential and refractory period in both atria and ventricles. Two adenosine receptors, A_1 and A_2, have been isolated which, when stimulated, prolong the refractory period in the atrioventricular node, slowing the heart, and causing arterial and coronary vasodilatation. The therapeutic serum concentration of digoxin ranges from 0.9–2.0 ng/l.

48. **The following reduce the MAC of volatile anaesthetic agents**
    A. Acidosis
    B. NMDA (*N*-methyl-D-aspartate) agonists
    C. Glutamate
    D. Dexmedetomidine
    E. Monoamine oxidase inhibitors

49. **The following statements concerning the analysis of vapours are true**
    A. Halothane absorbs ultraviolet light
    B. The Dräger Narkotest uses the principle that halothane absorbs infrared light to measure halothane concentrations
    C. The refractive index of a gas is the ratio of the velocity of light in a vacuum to the velocity of light in the gas
    D. Polarographic oxygen analysers measure the force experienced by oxygen molecules as they pass through a magnetic field
    E. The force experienced by oxygen molecules in a magnetic field is proportional to the partial pressure of oxygen

50. **The following statements regarding the full-term neonate are true**
    A. FRC is equivalent to adult values on a millilitre per kilogram basis
    B. The MAC of volatile anaesthetic agents is higher than in an infant of 6 months
    C. Systolic blood pressure is of the order of 95 mmHg
    D. A suitable endotracheal tube would have a 3.0 mm internal diameter
    E. The volume of distribution of bupivacaine is reduced

48. FFFTF

MAC is unaffected by acid–base status as well as the duration of anaesthesia and the gender of the patient. NMDA agonists stimulate glutamate-activated ion channels. As glutamate is an excitatory neurotransmitter in the CNS, NMDA agonists, as well as glutamate itself, will increase MAC. Ketamine and phencyclidine are NMDA antagonists and increase the potency of other anaesthetics. Dexmedetomidine, like clonidine, is an α_2-adrenergic agonist which increases the potency of anaesthetic drugs and produces sedation and analgesia.

49. TFTFT

Halothane absorbs ultraviolet light with maximum absorption in the region of 200 nm. The Dräger Narkotest measures the change in length of a piece of silicone rubber once halothane has been absorbed by it. Polarographic oxygen analysers, e.g. the Clark electrode, determine oxygen tension in the blood by measuring the current flow between two electrodes. Paramagnetic oxygen analysers measure the force exerted by oxygen molecules, which have been deflected by a magnetic field, on a nitrogen-filled dumb-bell.

50. TFFTT

Shortly after birth FRC rises to the equivalent of adult values on a millilitre per kilogram basis. Neonatal MAC is 15–25% below that of an infant aged 1–6 months. During the neonatal period the systolic blood pressure is of the order of 75 mmHg. Due to reduced plasma α_1 acid glycoprotein levels, the volume of distribution of bupivacaine is reduced and the proportion of free drug increased, leading to a greater risk of toxicity.

51. Regarding phaeochromocytoma
A. Ninety per cent of tumours are malignant
B. Malignant tumours never secrete dopamine
C. Adrenal tumours secrete both adrenaline and noradrenaline
D. Metaiodo-benzylguanidine has been used successfully to treat metastatic disease
E. Surgical cure only results in normotension in 15% of patients

52. The haemolytic uraemic syndrome is associated with
A. Anuria
B. Hemiparesis
C. Seizures
D. Acute pancreatitis
E. Coombs' positive haemolysis

53. Concerning non-steroidal anti-inflammatory drugs (NSAIDs)
A. Aspirin and diclofenac inhibit the production of prostaglandins and leukotrienes from arachidonic acid
B. The type I cyclo-oxygenase isoform (COX-1) is responsible for the production of inflammatory mediators from arachidonic acid
C. Aspirin is a specific COX-1 inhibitor
D. Diclofenac is a specific COX-2 inhibitor
E. Aspirin overdose can cause uncoupling of intracellular oxidative phosphorylation

51. FFTTF

Phaeochromocytomas can arise anywhere in the sympathetic chain but 90% occur in the adrenal medulla. Ten per cent are malignant. Malignant tumours may secrete dopamine. Adrenal tumours secrete both adrenaline and noradrenaline but tumours elsewhere secrete only noradrenaline. Surgery cures about 75% of the hypertension associated with the disease.

52. TTTTF

The haemolytic uraemic syndrome causes anuria in severe cases. CNS manifestations include hemiparesis and seizures. It is also associated with acute pancreatitis. Coombs' negative microangiopathic haemolysis can also occur.

53. FFTFT

NSAIDs inhibit cyclo-oxygenase with a fall in the production of the prostaglandin mediators of inflammation. Some NSAIDs, e.g. diclofenac and indomethacin but not aspirin, also inhibit lypoxygenase and reduce the production of leukotrienes, one of which, LTB4, is produced during inflammation. COX-1 produces prostaglandins responsible for functions such as vascular haemostasis. COX-2, which is induced during inflammation, produces prostaglandins, which mediate inflammation and cause fever and pain. NSAIDs differ in their selectivity between COX-1 and COX-2 isoforms. Aspirin, indomethacin and ibuprofen are more specific inhibitors of COX-1, while diclofenac, paracetamol and naproxen are equipotent against both isoforms.

54. Regarding the measurement of cardiac output
  A.   The direct Fick method involves measurement of the inspired oxygen concentration
  B.   When performing the thermal dilution method, a thermocouple measures the change in temperature in the pulmonary artery
  C.   Using the thermal dilution method, the lower the temperature of injectate, the greater the signal-to-noise ratio
  D.   The indirect Fick method involves the measurement of arteriovenous CO_2 difference
  E.   Both the thermal and dye dilution methods are prone to error because of significant recirculation of the indicator

55. Thiopentone and methohexitone
  A.   Methohexitone has twice the number of optical isomers that thiopentone has
  B.   Both cause significant sequelae when injected intra-arterially
  C.   Both contain a sulphur atom
  D.   Both may be administered rectally
  E.   Methohexitone is more potent than thiopentone

56. In accelerated hypertension
  A.   There is a diastolic blood pressure of $>120\,mmHg$ in adults
  B.   There is a grade III retinopathy
  C.   There may be hypertensive encephalopathy
  D.   There may be hypertensive heart failure
  E.   There may be progressive renal failure

54. FFTTF

The direct Fick method is based on the relationship $CO = VO_2/aO_2-vO_2$ where VO_2 = uptake of oxygen per minute and aO_2-vO_2 = arterial − venous oxygen difference. A spirometer is used to measure oxygen uptake and blood gas analysis measures the arteriovenous oxygen difference. A thermistor, not a thermocouple, is used to measure temperature change in the pulmonary artery. Only the dye dilution technique of cardiac output measurement is prone to error due to recirculation of the indicator.

55. TFFTT

Thiopentone has one asymmetric carbon atom but methohexitone has two. Although thiopentone produces severe adverse effects when injected intra-arterially, methohexitone causes mild discomfort only. Methohexitone does not possess a sulphur atom. Both thiopentone and methohexitone may be administered rectally. Methohexitone has approximately 2.7 times the anaesthetic potency of thiopentone.

56. TTTTT

The first two statements are requirements for the diagnosis to be made. Grade IV hypertensive retinopathy changes are the other manifestation that may be present. Hypertensive encephalopathy changes are diffuse and include coma, convulsions, focal defects, visual changes, blurred vision, headache and restlessness. Hypertensive retinopathy is difficult for anaesthetists to diagnose: grade I is arterial thickening and tortuous vessels, grade II is I + arteriovenous nipping, grade III is II + haemorrhages and exudates, and grade IV is III + papilloedema.

57. PEEP
- A. Has produced radiologically visible improvements in ARDS
- B. Effectiveness may be measured by increases in total static compliance
- C. Increases functional residual capacity
- D. May increase lung water
- E. Increases pulmonary vascular resistance

58. Ropivacaine
- A. Ropivacaine is a methyl homologue of bupivacaine
- B. Ropivacaine is less toxic than bupivacaine because it is less protein-bound
- C. The placental transfer of ropivacaine is less than that of lignocaine and similar to that of bupivacaine
- D. Ropivacaine causes local vasoconstriction
- E. The maximum safe dose of ropivacaine is 5 mg/kg

59. Pasteurization
- A. Is a form of sterilization
- B. Is more efficient than boiling
- C. Involves heating to 80°C for 10 min
- D. Involves heating to 70°C for 20 min
- E. Kills spores

60. Cardiomyopathy can be caused by
- A. Calcium overload
- B. Iron overload
- C. Phaeochromocytoma
- D. Amyloid
- E. Carcinoid syndrome

57. TTTTT

Studies using CT scanning have shown lung recruitment occurring with the application of PEEP. Total static compliance is a useful measure of the effectiveness of PEEP. Recruitment of collapsed alveoli increases functional residual capacity. PEEP does not reduce total lung water and may even increase it. Pulmonary vascular resistance is increased by PEEP.

58. FFTTF

Mepivacaine is a methyl homologue of bupivacaine. Ropivacaine is a propyl homologue of bupivacaine. Ropivacaine, like bupivacaine, is 95% protein-bound. It has the same relative toxicity as bupivacaine although cardiac side effects are less likely. The maximum safe dose is similar to bupivacaine, i.e. 2 mg/kg. Low placental transfer of bupivacaine and ropivacaine reflect extensive protein binding in the mother.

59. FFTTF

Pasteurization is a form of disinfection. It is less efficient than boiling. It consists of heating to 80°C for 10 min, or to 70°C for 20 min. It kills most infective organisms except spores.

60. FTTTT

There are three mechanisms of cardiomyopathy: dilatational, hypertrophic and restrictive. The main dilatational causes include alcohol, myocarditis, uraemia and sarcoid. The hypertrophic causes are idiopathic, glycogen storage diseases and muscular dystrophy. The restrictive causes include radiation, amyloid and carcinoid syndrome.

61. Cerebral vasospasm
  A. Has a sudden onset
  B. Risk is related to the amount of blood seen in the circle of Willis on CT scanning
  C. Risk is related to the degree of intraventricular haemorrhage
  D. Most commonly occurs 1–3 days following a subarachnoid haemorrhage
  E. Antifibrinolytic drugs increase the risk of vasospasm

62. The following statements concerning units of measurement are true
  A. $1\,N = 10\,000$ dynes
  B. $75\,mmHg = 10\,kPa$
  C. For a change in pH of one unit there is a hundred-fold change in hydrogen ion concentration
  D. The lux is the SI unit of luminous intensity
  E. The degree Celsius is a derived unit of temperature

63. The oxygen failure warning device
  A. Whistle lasts for 2 s
  B. The noise level 1 m away from the anaesthetic machine is 40 dB
  C. Whistle commences when oxygen pressure drops to 200 kPa
  D. At an oxygen pressure of 50 kPa the supply of anaesthetic gases cuts off
  E. Oxygen supply to the alarm arises downstream to the rotameters

64. Regarding hepatitis
  A. Hepatitis C is an RNA virus spread via the orofaecal route
  B. Blood transmission of hepatitis A occurs but is rare
  C. The incubation period of hepatitis A is 3–4 months
  D. In hepatitis A there is typically a leucopenia with a lymphocytosis
  E. The incubation period of hepatitis C is 2–8 weeks

61. FTFFT
Vasospasm has an insidious onset. The risk of vasospasm is related to the amount of blood visualized in the circle of Willis on CT scanning. Intraventricular haemorrhage does not increase the risk of vasospasm. Vasospasm most commonly occurs between days 4 and 14. Antifibrinolytic drugs reduce the risk of rebleeding but increase the risk of vasospasm.

62. FTFFT
One Newton force gives 1 kg an acceleration of $1 \, m/s^2$ or, in other words, 1 N gives 1000 g an acceleration of $100 \, cm/s^2$. As 1 dyne force gives 1 g an acceleration of $1 \, cm/s^2$, $1 \, N = 100\,000$ dyne. There is a ten-fold change in hydrogen ion concentration for each pH unit, e.g. pH $7.0 = [H^+]$ of $100 \, nmol/l$ whereas pH $8.0 = [H^+]$ of $10 \, nmol/l$. The candela (cd) is the SI unit of luminous intensity. Degrees Celsius = Kelvin (K) $- 273.15$.

63. FFFFF
The oxygen failure warning device has an auditory alarm which lasts for 7 s with a noise level of 60 dB at a distance of 1 m from the anaesthetic machine. The whistle commences when the supply pressure drops to 260 kPa and at around 200 kPa the supply of anaesthetic gases is cut off. The oxygen supply to the whistle originates upstream from the rotameters.

64. FTFTT
Hepatitis A is the form of hepatitis spread via the orofaecal route and it has an incubation period of 3–5 weeks. The viruses that cause hepatitis are hepatitis A, B, C, D, E, F and G, and others, termed non-A, non-B. Other viruses also cause it, including cytomegalovirus, Epstein–Barr virus and adenovirus. Toxoplasmosis (a protozoal infection) is clinically similar to viral hepatitis. It is not clear if hepatitis C and G cause an acute illness but the others do.

65. Hypothermia is associated with
  A.   Oliguria
  B.   Reduced sodium excretion
  C.   Acute pancreatitis
  D.   Forty per cent overall mortality
  E.   Reduced $P_{A-a}O_2$ gradient

66. Regarding the HELLP syndrome
  A.   The syndrome consists of haematuria, elevated liver enzymes and low platelets
  B.   It is diagnosed by an abnormal blood film and an elevated bilirubin with a normal lactic dehydrogenase
  C.   A macroangiopathic haemolysis occurs
  D.   A low platelet count in this syndrome is considered when the platelet count is $<100 \times 10^9/l$
  E.   Elevated liver enzymes result from periportal and focal parenchymal hepatic necrosis

67. Factors that alter the absorption of insulin include
  A.   Site of injection
  B.   Amount of subcutaneous fat
  C.   Temperature of insulin
  D.   Volume of insulin
  E.   Type of insulin

68. Artificial oxygen carriers
  A.   Perfluorocarbons are eliminated by metabolism
  B.   Perfluorocarbons are polymers
  C.   The terms first- and second-generation perfluorocarbons refer to the emulsifying agent used
  D.   The relationship between P_aO_2 and O_2 content of the blood is a linear one
  E.   Free haemoglobin solutions have a raised P_{50} value compared with haemoglobin in red blood cells

65. FFTFF

Hypothermia causes a diuresis that is associated with an increased sodium loss. Acute pancreatitis is a recognized complication of hypothermia. The overall mortality in hypothermia is 60%. Due to V/Q mismatch the $P_{A-a}O_2$ gradient increases.

66. FFFTT

The syndrome consists of haemolysis, elevated liver enzymes and low platelets. The haemolysis is microangiopathic and results from the passage of red cells through small blood vessels with damaged intimas. Large fibrinous deposits are seen in the sinusoids of the liver. An abnormal lactic dehydrogenase occurs. Symptoms usually occur before the 36th week but 30% occur in the post-partum period. Presenting symptoms include malaise, epigastric pain, nausea and vomiting, and flu-like symptoms. Signs include abdominal tenderness, oedema and weight gain. Recovery is slow and may take up to 11 days.

67. TTTTT

The other factor not included in the question is the amount of activity of the insulin. The absorption is slower if it is cold, inactive or given in a larger volume. A single injection of 48 units of insulin is more slowly absorbed than four injections of 12 units at different sites. Absorption is different depending on whether the arm, thigh or abdomen is used. The type of insulin determines its absorption and onset of action.

68. FFTTF

Perfluorocarbons are not metabolized but are rapidly phagocytosed by the reticuloendothelial cells and subsequently redistributed in the blood, transported to the lungs and exhaled. Perfluorocarbons consist of 8–10 carbon atoms. Due to an absence of 2,3-DPG, the P_{50} value of free haemoglobin is lower than that of intracellular haemoglobin.

69. Regarding intravenous opioid infusions
 A. The rate of recovery following a fentanyl infusion is primarily dependent on its elimination half-life ($t_{1/2}\beta$)
 B. The context sensitive half-time is the time for the effect-site concentration of a drug to fall by half following an infusion
 C. Following a 6 h infusion of alfentanil the effect-site concentration will fall by half after 2 h
 D. The elimination half-life of sufentanil is longer than that of alfentanil
 E. The time for the plasma concentration of remifentanil to fall by half is greater following a 6 h infusion than after a 1 h infusion

70. Referring to the measurement of temperature
 A. The relationship between the electromotive force (EMF) developed in a thermocouple and the temperature difference between its junctions is exponential
 B. Constantan is often used in thermocouples as it has a negligible temperature coefficient of resistance
 C. The Seebeck effect relates the change in electrical resistance that occurs in a metal to changing temperatures
 D. The resistance in a thermistor falls by 50% for each 20°C drop in temperature
 E. Thermistors are used in pulmonary artery catheters to measure cardiac output using the thermal dilution method

71. The following are important characteristics of peripheral nerve stimulators
 A. The electrical stimulus should be of 0.1–0.3 ms duration
 B. A current of 60–80 mA is required
 C. The waveform should be a monophasic square wave
 D. It should be able to produce a tetanic stimulus at 50 Hz
 E. It should deliver a train of four stimulus at 2 Hz

69. FTFTF
Following an infusion of the drug the rate of recovery
depends on the rate at which the drug diffuses from the
central compartment to the peripheral compartment, the
duration of the infusion, i.e. the quantity of drug infused, the
plasma concentration of the drug at the end of the infusion,
as well as the rate of metabolism and elimination of the
drug. The concentration of alfentanil falls by a half
50–60 min after stopping a 6 h alfentanil infusion. The
elimination half-lives of sufentanil and alfentanil are 165 and
90 min respectively. The plasma concentration of
remifentanil falls by half 5–6 min after stopping an infusion
regardless of its duration.

70. FTFFT
When the two junctions of a circuit composed of two
dissimilar metals are maintained at different temperatures an
EMF develops. This is a thermocouple and the effect is the
Seebeck effect. The relationship between the EMF and the
temperature difference between the junctions, one reference
and one measuring, is approximately parabolic. By choosing
particular metal pairings, e.g. copper and constantan (an
alloy of copper and nickel), the relationship becomes more
linear. The relationship between temperature and resistance
in a thermistor is exponential, resistance falling as
temperature rises. Therefore, resistance in a thermistor falls
by 50% for each 20°C increase in temperature.

71. TTTTT
A supra-maximal stimulus of 60–80 mA ensures the
depolarization of all nerve fibres being stimulated. The
waveform is monophasic so that the stimulator delivers a
constant current flowing over a specified interval.

72. The following statements regarding the stress response are true
A. Plasma free fatty acid levels increase
B. The circadian release of cortisol is abolished
C. Levels of angiotensin-converting enzyme are increased
D. Levels of cortisol correlate poorly with the degree of surgical trauma
E. The stress response is attenuated by morphine 4 mg/kg

73. Patients with uraemia have the following features
A. Cardiomyopathy
B. Peripheral neuropathy
C. Normal clotting
D. Pericarditis
E. Myopathy

74. Regarding calcium
A. Ionized plasma calcium increases with alkalosis
B. Calcium chloride solution 10% contains 10 mmol/10 ml of calcium ions
C. Calcium gluconate solution 10% contains 4.6 mmol/10 ml of calcium ions
D. Parathyroid hormone secretion is increased by hypocalcaemia and hypermagnesaemia
E. In hypoalbuminaemic patients, total plasma calcium readings are corrected by adding 0.04 mmol/l calcium for each 1 g/l albumin below 40 g/l

72. TFFFT

Secondary to lipolysis, plasma free fatty acid levels rise. The circadian release of cortisol is altered rather than abolished. Levels of angiotensin-converting enzyme are reduced. Levels of cortisol increase, correlating well with the degree of surgical trauma. A morphine dose of 4 mg/kg is required to attenuate the stress response.

73. TTFTT

The uraemic syndrome refers to two features of a patient with uraemia due to renal disease. Firstly the consequences of retaining excretory products are manifest, and secondly there is a group of signs and symptoms that are not easily explained but resolve after treatment. The clinical features include constitutional (malaise, lethargy), skin (pruritus, rashes), muscles (skeletal myopathy, cardiomyopathy, pericarditis, hypertension), endocrine (decreased sexual function), haematological (abnormal bleeding due to platelet dysfunction, impaired fibrin deposition, lowered factor VIII), and neurological (peripheral neuropathy and altered intellectual function).

74. FFFFF

As the hydrogen ion concentration falls, calcium binds more to albumin and plasma calcium falls. Ten per cent calcium chloride contains 6.8 mmol/10 ml, while 10% calcium gluconate contains 2.2–2.3 mmol/10 ml of calcium. Hypocalcaemia and hypomagnesaemia increase parathyroid hormone secretion. In hypoalbuminaemic patients, total plasma calcium readings are corrected by adding 0.02 mmol/l calcium for each 1 g/l albumin below 40 g/l.

75. Regarding the measurement of pH
    A.   A glass Ag/AgCl electrode is used in the pH electrode
    B.   A buffer is composed of a weak acid and its salt in addition to a strong base
    C.   The pH of blood falls as its temperature drops
    D.   The PCO_2 of blood can be determined once the pH is known
    E.   The pH electrode requires a battery

76. Butyrophenones
    A.   Act on GABA receptors
    B.   Are α-adrenergic receptor blockers
    C.   Are dopamine antagonists
    D.   Include droperidol
    E.   Have effects on the 5-HT receptor

77. Physiological effects of α_2 agonists include
    A.   Decreased intraocular pressure
    B.   Sedation, analgesia and anxiolysis
    C.   Salivation
    D.   Oliguria
    E. P_aCO_2 is unchanged

78. Regarding atopic eczema
    A.   Seventy-five per cent of the population have an atopic diathesis
    B.   Atopy means an inherited tendency to develop an altered state of immune reactivation with a type I hypersensitivity
    C.   An atopic diathesis is defined as a personal or first-degree family history of asthma, hayfever, eczema or conjunctivitis
    D.   Atopic patients have an elevated IgM
    E.   Patients with severe disease may be on cyclosporin A

75. TTFTF

In a pH meter the measuring electrode consists of an Ag/AgCl electrode within pH-sensitive glass, while the reference electrode uses mercury and a saturated solution of mercurous chloride or calomel. The pH of blood rises by 0.0147 for each degree Celsius fall in temperature. As there is a logarithmic relationship between blood pH and PCO_2, the PCO_2 of blood can be determined once the pH is known. The pH meter does not require a battery as it generates a potential that depends on the pH of the test solution.

76. TTTTF

Dopamine antagonism occurs at the chemoreceptor trigger zone, causing an anti-emetic effect.

77. TTFFF

Physiological effects of α_2 agonists include decreased intraocular pressure. In the CNS there is sedation, analgesia and anxiolysis. Gut effects include a dry mouth secondary to a decrease in vagal activity. α_2 agonists cause a diuresis. Following the administration of clonidine, P_aCO_2 rises secondary to a reduction in tidal volume.

78. FTTFT

Twenty-five per cent of the general population have an atopic diathesis and the IgE level is usually raised in these patients. Candidates should know how to define an atopic diathesis. Atopy is important as it can be brought into basic care topics such as anaphylaxis.

79. Peritoneal dialysis
   A.   Is associated with bradyarrhythmias
   B.   Utilization of 2–4 l of dialysate per day is normal
   C.   Caution should be exercised in the presence of intra-abdominal malignancy
   D.   The removal of large molecules is more effective when haemodialysis is used
   E.   Is contraindicated following intra-abdominal surgery

80. Concerning pulmonary artery occlusion pressure
   A.   Mitral stenosis causes underestimation of LVEDP
   B.   Mitral regurgitation causes underestimation of LVEDP
   C.   Dilated cardiomyopathy causes underestimation of LVEDV
   D.   Ischaemic heart disease causes underestimation of LVEDV
   E.   Aortic regurgitation causes overestimation of LVEDP

81. Duckett–Jones criteria for the diagnosis of rheumatic fever include
   A.   Huntington's chorea
   B.   Sydenham's chorea
   C.   Erythema nodosum
   D.   Small-joint polyarthritis
   E.   Subcutaneous nodules

79. TFFFF

Stretching of the peritoneum by fluid loads is arrhythmogenic. One to two litres are inserted during one dialysis cycle, totalling around 40 l/day. Intra-abdominal malignancy is an absolute contraindication to the use of peritoneal dialysis. Due to the large pore size in the peritoneal membrane, peritoneal dialysis is more effective than haemodialysis in removing large molecules. Previous abdominal surgery is not a contraindication to peritoneal dialysis.

80. FFTFF

Mitral valve disease leads to increased left atrial pressure (LAP). Pulmonary artery occlusion pressure (PAOP) therefore overestimates left ventricular end diastolic pressure (LVEDP). In a dilated cardiomyopathy the ventricle is very compliant and hence large rises in left ventricular end diastolic volume (LVEDV) will not be reflected in LVEDP. PAOP will therefore underestimate LVEDV. Ischaemic heart disease reduces ventricular compliance. PAOP will therefore overestimate LVEDV. With aortic regurgitation LAP does not reflect the LVEDP and therefore PAOP underestimates LVEDP.

81. FTFFT

Rheumatic fever is uncommon but still exists in poorer communities. The diagnosis is confirmed by having two or more major criteria or one major plus two or more minor criteria. The major criteria are large joint flitting arthritis, carditis, Sydenham's chorea (St. Vitus dance), erythema marginatum (a temporary raised rash on the trunk) and subcutaneous nodules. The minor criteria are previous rheumatic fever, arthralgia, fever, leucocytosis, raised ESR, raised ASO titre, and prolonged PR interval on the electrocardiograph.

82. In paracetamol poisoning
- A.   The clinical features can be delayed for up to 6 h
- B.   Early metabolic alkalosis can occur
- C.   Coma can occur early
- D.   Acetylcysteine lowers intracellular glutathione levels
- E.   The initial dose for acetylcysteine is 15 mg/kg over 15 min

83. Regarding ventilation of the lungs
- A.   The Manley ventilator is an example of a constant pressure-generating ventilator
- B.   Air flow rate falls exponentially during the inspiratory cycle when the lungs are ventilated by a constant pressure-generating ventilator
- C.   A ventilator which generates a constant flow has a high internal resistance
- D.   Using a pressure-generating ventilator the rate of lung inflation is dependent on the total compliance, the pulmonary resistance and the inflation pressure
- E.   A constant-flow generator has a high internal pressure source

84. The following treatments are appropriate in myxoedema coma
- A.   Intravenous T_4
- B.   Intravenous 10% dextrose
- C.   Fluid restriction
- D.   Rapid rewarming
- E.   IV hydrocortisone

82. FFFFF

Doses of >15 g of paracetamol can be fatal. Clinical features are often delayed for 18–24 h and signs of acute liver damage are not usually present for 36–48 h. If there is coma other drug ingestion should be suspected. An early metabolic acidosis occasionally occurs and this needs early treatment. Paracetamol is inactivated by hepatic conjugation – 85% is conjugated with glucuronide and sulphate and about 10% is oxidized to an intermediary (a hydroxylamine derivative) which then undergoes conjugation with glutathione. In overdose, glutathione becomes depleted and the object of treatment is to raise its levels. Acetylcysteine in an initial dose of 150 mg/kg over 15 min achieves this.

83. TTTFT

The weight on a Manley ventilator generates a constant pressure. The gas flow rate depends on the difference in pressure at any given time between the bellows of the ventilator and the patient's lungs. Initially this pressure difference is large but declines as the pressure in the lungs increases so that the flow rate falls exponentially. A constant flow generator has a very high internal pressure source and resistance so that the pressure generated in relation to the pressure change in the lungs during a respiratory cycle is very large. Therefore, the pressure difference between the pressure generator and the lungs, and therefore the flow, is constant throughout inflation. Using a pressure generator the time constant or rate of lung inflation = total compliance × pulmonary resistance, and is independent of inflation pressure.

84. FTTFF

Intravenous T_4 should be avoided as it may lead to cardiovascular collapse. T_3 via the oral or intravenous route should be administered. Hypoglycaemia will respond to intravenous glucose. Hyponatraemia responds to fluid restriction. Gradual rewarming is appropriate. Hydrocortisone should be administered intramuscularly.

85. Concerning the vaporization of halothane
   A.   The saturated vapour pressure of halothane at room temperature is 32 kPa
   B.   At an atmospheric pressure of 100 kPa and at room temperature, the partial pressure of halothane delivered from a halothane vaporizer set at 1% is 1 kPa
   C.   At an atmospheric pressure of 200 kPa and at room temperature, the partial pressure of halothane delivered from a halothane vaporizer set at 1% is 2 kPa
   D.   At an atmospheric pressure of 200 kPa, the setting of a halothane vaporizer should be reduced to 0.5% to achieve the same anaesthetic depth as a halothane vaporizer set at 1% at an atmospheric pressure of 100 kPa
   E.   The saturated vapour pressure of halothane falls if atmospheric pressure is increased

86. Regarding the transmission of pain impulses in the spinal cord
   A.   Glutamate, substance P and serotonin are excitatory substances released by $A\delta$ and C fibres in the dorsal horn of the spinal cord
   B. γ-amino-butyric acid (GABA) and acetylcholine inhibit pain transmission in the dorsal horn of the spinal cord
   C. μ-receptor stimulation by opioids causes hyperpolarization of pain afferent nerve endings, reducing neurotransmitter release in the dorsal horn of the spinal cord
   D. α_2-receptor agonists cause influx of chloride ions into $A\delta$ and C fibre afferent nerve endings, reducing neuro-transmitter release in the dorsal horn of the spinal cord
   E.   Ketamine is an *N*-methyl-D-aspartate (NMDA) receptor agonist

85. TTFFF

Saturated vapour pressure is dependent only on ambient temperature, rising as temperature increases. It is unaffected by ambient pressure. 32 kPa, the SVP of halothane at room temperature, represents 32% of the atmospheric pressure at 100 kPa and 16% of the atmospheric pressure at 200 kPa. Therefore, at 200 kPa there is a halving of the percentage of halothane in the vaporization chamber and consequently a halving of the output of halothane measured at 200 kPa, so that a vaporizer set at 1% will actually deliver 0.5% at 200 kPa. It follows that the partial pressure of halothane delivered from a vaporizer set at 1% at an atmospheric pressure of 200 kPa is 0.5% × 200 kPa = 1 kPa. This is the same as the partial pressure delivered from a vaporizer set at 1% at an atmospheric pressure of 100 kPa, i.e. 1% × 100 kPa = 1 kPa. As it is the partial pressure of halothane and **not** the percentage that determines the depth of anaesthesia, the vaporizer setting should remain at 1% whatever the ambient atmospheric pressure.

86. FTTFF

Aspartate, calcitonin and possibly NMDA, as well as glutamate and substance P, are excitatory substances released by Aδ and C fibres. Serotonin, however, as well as GABA, acetylcholine, α_2-receptor agonists and endogenous opioids are inhibitory influences in the dorsal horn of the spinal cord. Both μ and α_2 receptor stimulation causes hyperpolarization of presynaptic nerve endings in the dorsal horn by increasing the efflux of potassium ions. GABA causes presynaptic hyperpolarization by increasing the influx of negatively charged chloride ions. Hyperpolarization of presynaptic Aδ and C fibres in the dorsal horn reduces neurotransmitter release. Ketamine is an NMDA antagonist.

87. **Concerning adverse reactions and anaesthesia**
    A. Mast cell degranulation is favoured by a reduced intracellular cGMP
    B. Morphine is a common trigger of anaphylaxis
    C. Blood transfusion incompatibility reactions are an example of a type III hypersensitivity reaction
    D. Prognosis in anaphylaxis is worsened by the presence of epidural anaesthesia
    E. Reaction to thiopentone usually follows multiple previous exposures

88. **Regarding the drug therapy of diabetes mellitus**
    A. Tolbutamide may act by increasing secretion of insulin by the pancreas
    B. Metformin may increase insulin binding to receptors and also impair gluconeogenesis
    C. Sulphonylureas are contraindicated in porphyria
    D. Chlorpropamide can cause lactic acidosis
    E. Metformin has a mild anorexic effect which causes weight loss

89. **Amniotic fluid embolism**
    A. Has an average incidence of 1 in 200 000
    B. Has a 50% mortality
    C. The presence of fetal squames in the maternal circulation is pathognomonic
    D. Is associated with the intra-uterine injection of hypertonic saline
    E. Bronchospasm is often a presenting feature

90. **Glycine when used as irrigation for transurethral resection**
    A. May cause visual disturbance
    B. Releases ADH
    C. Produces an osmotic diuresis
    D. Is isotonic with plasma
    E. Dissipates electric current from the resectoscope

87. **FFFTT**
Increased intracellular levels of cGMP favour mast cell degranulation. Morphine is extremely rarely found to be the cause of anaphylactic reactions. Blood transfusion incompatibility reactions are an example of type II hypersensitivity reactions. The presence of epidural anaesthesia worsens the prognosis in anaphylactic reactions. Reaction to thiopentone is characterized by multiple previous uneventful exposures.

88. **TTTFT**
Metformin causes lactic acidosis. Of the sulphonylureas, chlorpropamide has the longest half-life. It is taken once daily and runs the biggest risk of causing delayed hypoglycaemia under general anaesthesia.

89. **FFFTF**
Amniotic fluid embolism has an average incidence of 1 in 20 000. The mortality rate is 86%. Historically it was thought that fetal squames in the maternal venous system were pathognomonic, but these are present during normal labour and delivery. Amniotic fluid embolism has followed the intra-uterine injection of hypertonic saline during abortion. Bronchospasm is rarely a feature of amniotic fluid embolism

90. **TTTFF**
Glycine directly affects the central nervous system, causing visual disturbances and releasing ADH. Ten per cent of absorbed glycine is excreted in the urine causing an osmotic diuresis. Glycine is presented as a 1.5% solution which is hypotonic to plasma. It is used in preference to electrolyte solutions as it does not dissipate electric current from the resectoscope.

Paper 4

1. **Characteristic features of pre-renal failure include**
   A.   High urinary sodium concentration
   B.   Low urinary urea concentration
   C.   High urine osmolality
   D.   Urine:plasma osmolality ratio of 2:1
   E.   Proteinuria is present

2. **Regarding local anaesthetic block of the foot at the ankle**
   A.   The tibial nerve (L5–S1) is blocked at the level of the medial malleolus as it passes posterior to the tibial artery
   B.   The tibial nerve supplies the medial aspect of the sole of the foot
   C.   The sural nerve is formed from branches of the saphenous nerve and supplies the heel and lateral side of the foot
   D.   The superficial peroneal nerve supplies the skin over the area of the first and second toes
   E.   The cutaneous branch of the common peroneal nerve supplies the medial aspect of the ankle joint

3. **Regarding vaporizers**
   A.   The Oxford Miniature Vaporizer (OMV) is a plenum vaporizer
   B.   The EMO vaporizer is surrounded by a jacket containing ethylene glycol which acts as a heat reservoir
   C.   The EMO vaporizer is not temperature-compensated
   D.   The EMO vaporizer delivers dangerously high concentrations of ether when used as a continuous-flow plenum-type vaporizer
   E.   The OMV can be used with halothane and ether

1. **FFTTF**

   The characteristic features of prerenal failure include a concentrated urine with a low sodium and a high urea content. The urine:plasma osmolality ratio is of the order of 2:1. Proteinuria is absent.

2. **TTFFF**

   The sural nerve (L5–S2) is formed from branches of the tibial and common peroneal nerves and supplies the heel and lateral side of the foot. The deep peroneal nerve supplies skin over the first and second toes, while the superficial peroneal nerve supplies skin over the dorsum of the foot and is blocked by subcutaneous infiltration from the lateral malleolus to the anterior aspect of the tibia. The saphenous nerve, which is the terminal branch of the femoral nerve, supplies the medial aspect of the ankle joint.

3. **FFFFF**

   The EMO and OMV vaporizers are both draw-over vaporizers. A water jacket surrounds the EMO vaporizers providing a source of heat, while a set of bellows filled with ether vapour acts as a temperature compensation valve at the chamber outlet. As the temperature falls the bellows contract and open the valve. When used as a plenum vaporizer, the EMO delivers a lower percentage of anaesthetic than indicated. The OMV has a small water reservoir that acts as a heat sink, but no thermo-compensation. It can be used with halothane, trilene or enflurane.

4. Concerning the barbiturates
- A. Both isomers of thiopentone penetrate the CNS to a similar degree
- B. The addition of sulphur to the barbiturate ring increases its duration of action
- C. The hypnotic effects are terminated by metabolism
- D. Increasing lipophilicity increases duration of action
- E. They are useful in protecting the brain following cardiac arrest

5. ECT and anaesthesia
- A. Current applied to initiate a seizure is in the form of a sine wave
- B. To be effective the seizure must last for >30 s
- C. Asystole may occur as a direct result of ECT
- D. Bradycardia should be pretreated with atropine
- E. ECT causes a rise in intracranial pressure

6. Drugs that may precipitate an acute attack of porphyria include
- A. Thiopentone
- B. Chlordiazepoxide
- C. Phenytoin
- D. Sulphonamides
- E. Chloramphenicol

4. TFFFF

Although the L-isomer of thiopentone has twice the potency of the D-isomer, both penetrate the CNS to a similar degree. The addition of sulphur to the barbiturate ring increases the speed of onset and reduces the duration of action. The hypnotic effects of the barbiturates are terminated by redistribution. Increasing the lipophilicity reduces the duration of action of the barbiturates. Barbiturates have not been found effective in brain protection following a global cerebral insult.

5. FTTFT

The current applied to initiate the seizure is in the form of a square wave. To be therapeutic the seizure must last more than 30 seconds. Parasympathetic activation can cause asystole. Atropine crosses the blood–brain barrier and may synergize with anticholinergic medication causing post ECT confusion. ECT causes initial cerebrovascular vasoconstriction followed by a sustained increase in metabolism and flow, raising intracranial pressure.

6. TTTTT

No one can remember every drug that is safe or unsafe. Even examiners have to look them up, but the five mentioned in the question are the ones that all anaesthetists should know. Precipitating factors for an acute attack include alcohol, synthetic oestrogens and progesterones, meprobamate, and a weight-reducing diet (everyone's on a diet!). Tell the examiner that you would seek advice and look up safe drugs to give.

7. The causes of hypercalcaemia include
A. Thiazide diuretics
B. Lithium
C. Aminophylline
D. Conn's syndrome
E. Phaeochromocytoma

8. Regarding tetanus
A. Tetanus toxin causes haemolysis
B. Tetanus toxin is an endotoxin
C. Sympathetic overactivity may lead to sudden death
D. Multiplication of *Clostridium tetani* occurs in the anterior horn cell
E. In the absence of hypoxia, consciousness is preserved

9. The following statements regarding neuromuscular junction monitoring are true
A. A phase II block exhibits fade in response to a train of four stimulus
B. The single-twitch response only falls once 60% of acetylcholine receptors are blocked
C. The fourth twitch of a train of four stimulus disappears when 60–65% of acetylcholine receptors are blocked
D. The ability to sustain a head lift for 5 s correlates with 33% or less occupancy of receptors by neuromuscular blocking agents
E. When 90–95% of acetylcholine receptors are blocked, there is no response to a train of four stimulus

7. TTTFT

Conn's syndrome does not cause hypercalcaemia.
Hypercalcaemia is caused in the following conditions:
endocrine (hypercalcaemia, thyrotoxicosis, Addison's disease,
phaeochromocytoma), malignancy, drugs (vitamin D and A
intoxication, milk-alkali syndrome, thiazides, lithium,
aminophylline), prolonged immobilization, renal failure,
granulomatous disease (including sarcoidosis, tuberculosis),
and familial.

8. TFTFT

Clostridium tetani produces a protein exotoxin, which
consists of two components: tetanospasmin, which is
responsible for neurological manifestations, and tetanolysin
which lyses erythrocytes. Tetanus is extremely rare in the
UK. A common cause of death is cardiac arrest due to
sympathetic overactivity. *Clostridium tetani* remains in the
wound site. Consciousness is preserved in the absence of
hypoxia.

9. TFFTT

The single twitch response falls when 75% of receptors are
blocked and it disappears when 90–95% are occupied. The
fourth twitch of a train of four disappears when 75–80% of
receptors are occupied, the third at 85% occupancy, the
second at 85–90% occupancy and the first twitch is lost when
90–95% of receptors are blocked. The head lift test is the
most sensitive clinical measure of adequate reversal from
neuromuscular blockade. In comparison, patients with
adequate tidal volumes may still have 80% of their
acetylcholine receptors blocked.

10. **Regarding the apparatus used in the direct measurement of intra-arterial blood pressure**
    A. The natural frequency of the catheter transducer system is the frequency at which it resonates
    B. The natural frequency of the catheter transducer system is proportional to the diameter of the catheter lumen
    C. Following a high-pressure flush of the manometer tubing an overdamped system oscillates before settling to baseline
    D. In both overdamped and underdamped systems the mean arterial pressure is relatively accurate
    E. The natural frequency of the monitoring system is dependent on the square root of its compliance

11. **Myasthenia gravis**
    A. There is increased sensitivity to depolarizing agents
    B. There is a reduced tendency to develop phase II block
    C. Cholinesterase inhibitors are useful in severe disease
    D. Steroids improve the condition in 50% of cases
    E. Complete thymectomy is best achieved via the transcervical approach

12. **Regarding diabetic glomerulopathy**
    A. The risk of glomerulopathy increases with the duration of the diabetes
    B. It is less common in insulin-dependent diabetics
    C. Hypertension is a late feature
    D. The progression of the renal failure is unaffected by the quality of glycaemic control
    E. It usually occurs in isolation from other diabetic complications

10. TTFTT

The natural frequency of the measuring apparatus is the frequency at which it resonates and amplifies the signals it receives. The natural frequency is proportional to the diameter of the manometer tubing and inversely proportional to the density of the fluid inside the tubing and the square roots of both the tubing length and compliance of the whole measuring system. An underdamped system continues to oscillate for 3–4 cycles after a high-pressure flush whereas an overdamped system drifts slowly to baseline without oscillating. An underdamped system overestimates the systolic and underestimates the diastolic blood pressure, while exactly the opposite is true of an overdamped system. In both cases, however, the mean blood pressure is relatively accurate.

11. FFFFF

Myasthenia gravis is characterized by a resistance to depolarizing neuromuscular blockers, with increased likelihood of phase II block. Cholinesterase inhibitors represent symptomatic therapy and are only useful in mild disease. Steroids improve the condition in 80% of cases. Complete thymectomy is not possible via the transcervical approach. To attempt complete removal, the trans-sternal approach is advisable.

12. TFFFF

Diabetic glomerulopathy affects about 30% of people who have been diabetics for more than 20 years. It is more common in insulin-dependent diabetics. It is usually associated with patients who have other diabetic complications (peripheral neuropathy, atherosclerosis). It will finally lead to end-stage renal failure if left untreated. Hypertension is an early sign and will accelerate the progression of failure. Treatment of the hypertension is effective control, with ACE inhibitors being especially beneficial because they lower intra-glomerular pressure. Good glycaemic control will also slow the disease.

13. The intra-aortic balloon pump
   A.   Inflates synchronously with the 'R' wave on the ECG
   B.   Decreases afterload
   C.   Increases coronary blood flow
   D.   Lowers left ventricular wall tension
   E.   Is usually inserted percutaneously via the femoral vein

14. Regarding plasma tonicity
   A.   Osmolarity is defined as the number of osmoles of solute per kilogram of solvent
   B.   The freezing point of an aqueous solution rises by $1.86°C$ per osmole of solute
   C.   Osmoreceptors are located in the left atrium and the supraoptic nuclei of the hypothalamus
   D.   The sensation of thirst is stimulated by an increase in plasma osmolarity of 4 mosmol/l
   E.   Angiotensin II stimulates thirst receptors in the hypothalamus

15. Brachial plexus blocks
   A.   The most rapid onset occurs with the interscalene block
   B.   Axillary nerve block is associated with incomplete analgesia of the medial part of the arm
   C.   Interscalene block is associated with incomplete analgesia of the thumb
   D.   Supraclavicular block is associated with the most complete analgesia of the arm
   E.   Supraclavicular block is always associated with immediate onset pneumothorax

13. FTTTF

The intra-aortic balloon pump deflates at the onset of systole – the 'R' wave on the ECG. It reduces afterload, which has the effect of increasing coronary blood flow and lowering myocardial wall tension. It is usually inserted percutaneously via the femoral artery.

14. FFFTT

Osmolarity is the number of osmoles of solute per litre of solution. Osmolality is the number of osmoles per kilogram of solvent. The freezing point of an aqueous solution falls by 1.86°C per osmole of solute, which is why ice melts when sprinkled with salt. There are no osmoreceptors in the left atrium although they are present in the supraoptic nuclei. Stretch receptors in the left atrium respond to changes in intravascular volume. Thirst receptors in the hypothalamus respond to an increase in plasma sodium of 2 mEq/1 and potassium loss, as well as to angiotensin II and an increase in plasma osmolality. (They are also stimulated by the sight of a hostelry.) Activation of the thirst centre results in release of ADH.

15. FFFTF

The most rapid onset is associated with the supraclavicular approach. With an axillary nerve block the musculocutaneous nerve is often missed leading to incomplete analgesia of the lateral part of the arm. The interscalene block is associated with failure to block the ulnar nerve. This leads to incomplete block of the little and ring fingers. Supraclavicular block is associated with most complete analgesia of the arm. Pneumothoracies occurring with the supraclavicular approach can be delayed in onset, occurring up to 24 h later.

16. **Regarding fulminant hepatic failure**
    A. It can follow acute fatty liver of pregnancy
    B. It is defined as hepatic encephalopathy occurring within 18 weeks of the onset of symptoms in a person with or without previous liver disease
    C. Ninety-five per cent of cases are due to paracetamol overdose or viral hepatitis
    D. A low alkaline phosphatase and very high serum transferases may indicate Gilbert's disease
    E. Factor V levels or prothrombin time are the best indicators of prognosis

17. **Regarding post-dural puncture headache**
    A. It can be associated with a transient hearing loss
    B. It relates to the diameter of the needle involved
    C. In 85% of patients the headache is diffuse and radiates to the neck
    D. It can be associated with tinnitus
    E. It can be associated with ptosis

18. **The following drugs are useful in the management of Guillain–Barré syndrome**
    A. Atropine
    B. β-blockers
    C. Quinine
    D. Methadone
    E. Steroids

19. **The following statements about inhaled nitric oxide are true**
    A. Inhaled nitric oxide will decrease pulmonary vascular resistance in normal subjects
    B. Nitric oxide increases platelet aggregation
    C. Nitric oxide is synthesized from L-arginine
    D. Physiological effects are mediated by decreasing intracellular cyclic GMP
    E. An appropriate concentration is 200–400 p.p.m.

16. TFTTT

The definition is important. Fulminant hepatic failure is hepatic encephalopathy occurring within 8 weeks of the onset of symptoms in a person with a previously normal liver. Other rare causes are drug induced (halothane), sepsis and malignancy. Confusion, drowsiness and coma occur and hypoglycaemia presents as the condition worsens. Multisystem failure eventually occurs.

17. TTFTF

There is an association between the headache, the rate of cerebrospinal fluid loss, the size of the dural breech and the diameter and shape of the needle used. In 50% of patients the headache is localized to the frontal area, in 25% it is localized to the occiput, and in the remaining 25% the headache is diffuse and radiates to the neck. It is always postural. It is associated with auditory (tinnitus, hearing loss, dizziness) and visual (blurred or double vision, photophobia) symptoms. Sixth cranial nerve palsies occur.

18. TTTTF

Both atropine and β-blockers are useful in the management of autonomic instability. Quinine and methadone have been used to control limb pain. Steroids do not favourably alter the course of Guillain–Barré syndrome.

19. FFTFF

Inhaled nitric oxide has no effect on the normal non-constricted pulmonary circulation. Nitric oxide inhibits platelet aggregation by increasing platelet cyclic guanosine monophosphate. Nitric oxide synthetase utilizes L-arginine and oxygen to produce nitric oxide. Vasodilatation due to nitric oxide is mediated by increasing cyclic guanosine monophosphate levels. At levels >200 p.p.m. nitric oxide is toxic.

20. The following are included in Goldman's criteria of cardiac risk factors associated with non-cardiac surgery
   A.   Mitral stenosis
   B.   Male gender
   C.   Jugular venous distension
   D.   Major orthopaedic surgery
   E.   Age >60

21. The following are basic SI units
   A.   Volt
   B.   Mole
   C.   Newton
   D.   Pascal
   E.   Joule

20. FFTFF

There are nine independent risk factors for life-threatening complications during non-cardiac surgery as classified by Goldman:

(1) Pre-operative third heart sound or jugular venous distension.
(2) MI in the preceding 6 months.
(3) More than five premature ventricular contractions per minute recorded pre-operatively.
(4) Cardiac rhythm other than sinus.
(5) Age over 70.
(6) Intraperitoneal, intrathoracic or aortic surgery.
(7) Emergency operation.
(8) Significant aortic stenosis.
(9) Poor general health.

21. FTFFF

There are seven basic SI units: metre, second, kilogram, ampere, kelvin, candela and mole. All other units are derived.

1 newton (N) is the force required to accelerate a mass of 1 kg by $1 \, m/s^2$.

1 pascal (pa) of pressure $= 1 \, N/m^2$.

1 joule (j) is the work done when the point of application of a force of 1 newton moves 1 metre in the direction of the force, i.e. 1 joule = 1 newton × 1 metre.

1 volt is the potential difference between two points when 1 joule of work is done per coulomb of electricity passing from one point to another. (1 coulomb is the amount of charge passing any point in an electrical circuit in 1 second when a current of 1 ampere is flowing.)

22. Concerning viscosity
  A. Laminar flow rate is inversely proportional to viscosity
  B. Reynold's number is inversely proportional to viscosity
  C. The SI unit of viscosity is the tesla
  D. Compared to water, the relative viscosity of plasma is 3.5
  E. Blood viscosity increases markedly in blood vessels which are <0.3 mm in diameter

23. Halothane
  A. Lowers left atrial pressure
  B. Reduces splanchnic blood flow
  C. Reduces renal blood flow
  D. Has a higher boiling point than enflurane
  E. Is stable in sunlight

24. The Tec 6 vaporizer
  A. Is electronically heated to 30°C
  B. Can only be used with desflurane
  C. Mixing of the volatile agent and carrier gas occurs in the vaporizing chamber
  D. Is refilled using the Fraser–Sweatman filling system
  E. The system is pressurized

22. TTFFF

The SI unit of viscosity is the poise and is the tendency of fluids to resist flow.

Laminar flow = $P\pi r^4/8\eta l$

– where P is the pressure gradient along the tube, r is the radius of the tube, l is the length of the tube, η is the viscosity of the fluid in the tube.

Reynold's number (Re) predicts when flow will become turbulent. If Re is greater than 2000 flow will be turbulent whereas if Re is lower than 2000 flow will be laminar.

$Re = \rho v d/\eta$

– where η is the viscosity of the fluid, ρ is the density of the fluid, v is the velocity of the fluid, d is the diameter of the tube.

The relative viscosity of plasma is 1.5 while that of whole blood is 3.5. As blood is a non-newtonian fluid its viscosity drops markedly in blood vessels with a diameter of less than 0.3 mm. This results in a higher flow rate in these vessels.

23. FTTFF

The myocardial depressant effect of halothane leads to an increased left ventricular end diastolic pressure that in turn leads to an increased left atrial pressure. Both splanchnic and renal blood flow are reduced by halothane. The boiling point of enflurane is 56.5°C and the boiling point of halothane is 50.2°C. Halothane is unstable in sunlight which is why it is stored in a brown bottle.

24. FTFFT

The Tec 6 vaporizer is electronically heated and pressurized. It may only be used with desflurane that is heated to 39°C. Mixing of desflurane vapour and the carrier gas occurs at the outlet of the vaporizer. The Fraser–Sweatman filling system is not used with the Tec 6.

25. Regarding phaeochromocytoma
   A.   It can occur as part of multiple endocrine neoplasia
   B.   Multiple endocrine neoplasia type 2 can be familial
        (autosomal-dominant inheritance)
   C.   Fifty per cent of these patients have von
        Recklinghausen's disease
   D.   Fifty per cent of tumours are within the adrenal medulla
   E.   Patients with multiple endocrine neoplasia type 3 may
        have mucosal neuromas on the lips and tongue

26. Concerning subarachnoid haemorrhage
   A.   Sex distribution is equal
   B.   Systemic hypertension is not a risk factor
   C.   Incidence is reduced in the immediate post-partum
        period
   D.   Most commonly occurs between the ages 40 and 60
        years
   E.   Rupture of Charcot–Buchard aneurysms is implicated

27. Acute epiglottitis
   A.   May have a viral aetiology
   B.   The peak incidence is from ages 1–4 years
   C.   There is an equal sex distribution
   D.   Nebulized adrenaline is useful
   E.   Aphonia is a feature

28. In paracetamol poisoning
   A.   Doses of >15 g can be fatal in adults
   B.   Normally paracetamol is inactivated in the liver by
        oxidation
   C.   In therapeutic doses, 85% is oxidized with gluconuride
        and sulphate
   D.   In therapeutic doses, approximately 10% is oxidized and
        then conjugated with glutathione
   E.   The hydroxylamine metabolite directly affects both liver
        and renal cells, leading to acute hepatic and renal
        tubular necrosis

25. TTFFT

Phaeochromocytoma is rare with a prevalence of about 0.2% of hypertensive patients. About 5% are inherited. Approximately 5% of patients have von Recklinghausen's disease. Patients with hereditary cerebellar ataxia (Sturge–Weber disease), and cerebello-retinal haemangio-blastomatosis (von Hippel–Lindau syndrome) also have a greater than expected prevalence of the disease. Phaeochromocytomas can lie anywhere in the sympathetic chain but 90% occur in the adrenal medulla.

26. FTFTF

Subarachnoid haemorrhage (SAH) has a male to female ratio of 1.6:1.0. Systemic hypertension is not a risk factor for SAH but its presence worsens the prognosis. SAH has an increased incidence during pregnancy and the puerperium. The most common age group is 40–60 years. Charcot–Buchard aneurysms are associated with intracerebral haemorrhage.

27. TFFFT

Acute epiglottitis is usually caused by the bacteria *haemophilus influenza* but viruses can cause it. The most common virus implicated is the parainfluenzae myxovirus. The peak age incidence is 2–7 years with a slightly increased incidence in males. The use of nebulized adrenaline may make the condition worse. Dysphonia progressing to aphonia is a feature.

28. TFFTT

Indeed 30 tablets of paracetamol can be fatal in adults. The drug is conjugated in the liver. In therapeutic doses 10% is oxidized to the intermediary hydroxylamine derivative which is then conjugated with glutathione. As glutathione stores are depleted the intermediary is built up causing liver and kidney toxicity.

29. The first rib
  A. Possesses a single articular facet on its head
  B. Scalenus medius inserts into the scalene tubercle
  C. The sympathetic trunk lies lateral to its neck
  D. The lower cords of the brachial plexus pass anterior to scalenus medius
  E. Serratus anterior is attached to the lateral margin of the 1st rib

30. Regarding coagulation of blood
  A. The partial thromboplastin time (PTT) is normal in 40–50% of patients with disseminated intravascular coagulation (DIC)
  B. The normal activated clotting time (ACT) is 90–120 s
  C. Subcutaneous vitamin K takes 48 h to reverse the effects of warfarin
  D. D-dimers are formed as a result of the breakdown of fibrin by plasmin
  E. Cryoprecipitate is used in the treatment of antithrombin III deficiency

31. The following prolong the QT interval of the ECG
  A. Hypocalcaemia
  B. Hypermagnesaemia
  C. Amiodarone
  D. Head injury
  E. Tricyclic antidepressants

32. Suxamethonium
  A. Muscle pains are unrelated to the extent of the surgery
  B. Peak rise in intraocular pressure occurs at 1–2 min
  C. Neostigmine does not affect the duration of the block
  D. MAOI therapy may increase the duration of the block
  E. Does not produce active metabolites

29. TFFFT
The 1st rib possesses a single articular facet at its head, articulating with the body of T1. Scalenus anterior inserts into the scalene tubercle. The sympathetic trunk lies medial to the 1st rib. The lower trunks of the brachial plexus cross the 1st rib. The serratus anterior is attached to the lateral margin of the 1st rib.

30. TTFFF
PTT is increased in only 50–60% of patients with DIC while the prothrombin time (PT) is elevated in 75%. The effects of warfarin are reversed by subcutaneous vitamin K within 6–24 hours. In an emergency, fresh frozen plasma (FFP) should be given. D-dimers are formed when fibrinogen is converted to cross-linked fibrin by the action of thrombin, whereas fibrin degradation products (FDP) are produced when plasmin breaks down fibrin clots. FFP is used in the treatment of antithrombin III deficiency.

31. TFTTT
The causes of a prolonged QT interval are:
(1) Antiarrhythmic drugs which prolong repolarization, e.g. quinidine, procainamide, sotolol and amiodarone.
(2) Other drugs, e.g. tricyclic antidepressants, lithium and phenothiazenes.
(3) Electrolyte disturbance, e.g. hypokalaemia, hypocalcaemia and hypomagnesaemia.
(4) CNS disorders, e.g. head injury, subarachnoid haemorrhage.
(5) Cardiac cause, e.g. ischaemia and myocarditis.

32. FFFTF
Muscle pains are more prominent following minor surgery. The rise in intraocular pressure peaks at 2–4 min. Prior administration of neostigmine prolongs the action of suxamethonium due to inhibition of pseudocholinesterase. Phenelzine, an MAOI, reduces pseudocholinesterase activity by up to 40%. Succinyl monocholine has weak neuromuscular blocking activity.

33. Neoplastic causes of lower back pain include
A.   Multiple myeloma
B.   Secondary carcinoma of the breast
C.   Secondary astrocytoma
D.   Secondary carcinoma of the prostate
E.   Secondary carcinoma of the thyroid

34. The following are absolute contraindications to the placement of a pulmonary artery catheter
A.   Right atrial myxoma
B.   Pulmonary stenosis
C.   Coagulopathy
D.   A permanent pacemaker, inserted within the last 6 weeks
E.   Tetralogy of Fallot

35. *Pneumocystis carinii* pneumonia in patients with AIDS
A.   Has a rapid onset
B.   Pleural effusions are a feature
C.   Treatment involves co-trimoxazole 120 mg/kg/day
D.   Steroids do not improve survival
E.   The institution of mechanical ventilation produces a large rise in P_aO_2

33. **TTFTT**

Back pain is a common referral symptom to chronic pain clinics. Most patients present with the correct diagnosis but sometimes the cause needs the diagnostic skills of the anaesthetist. It can be differentiated into the following causes: mechanical, neoplastic, inflammatory, infective, metabolic and referred. The malignant causes are primary bone tumours, secondary bone tumours (breast, bronchus, kidney, thyroid, prostate and bowel), myeloma, and the spinal cord and its coverings. The infective causes are rare but include *Mycobacterium tuberculosis*, *Salmonella*, and *Brucella*.

34. **TTFFT**

Right atrial myxoma, pulmonary stenosis and tetralogy of Fallot are absolute contraindications to the placement of a pulmonary artery catheter. In tetralogy of Fallot the catheter may cause severe cyanosis by eliciting spasm of the right ventricular outflow tract. A pacemaker inserted within the previous 6 weeks represents a relative contraindication, as the catheter may dislodge the wires.

35. **FFTFF**

Pneumocystis carinii pneumonia in patients with AIDS has an insidious onset. Pleural effusions are not typically a feature. The treatment involves high-dose co-trimoxazole (120mg/kg/24h). Steroids have been shown to increase survival and reduce the incidence of respiratory failure. Mechanical ventilation produces only modest increases in P_aO_2.

36. **Concerning immunoglobulins**
    A.   Immunoglobulins are used to treat digoxin toxicity
    B.   IgE causes histamine release
    C.   IgA is involved with complement fixation
    D.   IgM is the most abundant immunoglobulin in the plasma
    E.   Anaesthetic drug reactions are due to IgG-mediated complement fixation

37. **Etomidate**
    A.   Increases ACTH levels
    B.   Is water-soluble
    C.   Is 90% protein-bound
    D.   The (−) isomer has hypnotic properties
    E.   Reduces intracranial pressure

38. **Regarding the spinal cord**
    A.   The anterior spinal artery originates from the vertebral artery
    B.   Following spinal cord injury, denervated muscle responds with proliferation of extra-junctional acetylcholine receptors after 72 h
    C.   Autonomic hyper-reflexia occurs immediately after injury to the spinal cord
    D.   The maximal autonomic hyper-reflexic response in a patient with spinal cord injury occurs following stimulation of the anorectal area
    E.   The artery of Adamkiewicz supplies the lumbar region of the spinal cord

39. **The following statements regarding lung volumes in adults are true**
    A.   The normal FEV_1 is 1–2 l
    B.   Residual volume (RV) is reduced in asthmatic patients
    C.   Total lung capacity (TLC) is increased in emphysema
    D.   Diffusion capacity is normal in emphysema
    E.   The normal residual volume is 1–2 l

36. TTFFT

Digoxin-specific antibodies derived from sheep immunoglobulins are used to treat toxicity. IgG is the most abundant immunoglobulin and is involved, as is IgM, with complement fixation. IgE is on the surface of mast cells and causes histamine release. IgA is secreted from endothelium, e.g. gut. IgD is involved with antigen recognition by lymphocytes.

37. TFFFT

ACTH rises in response to the inhibition of steroid synthesis by etomidate. Etomidate is not water soluble and is 75% protein bound. The (+) isomer is active while the (−) isomer has no hypnotic activity. Etomidate lowers intracranial pressure.

38. TFFTT

Extra acetylcholine receptors are generated within 48–72 h of spinal cord injury. The peak release of potassium following suxamethonium is approximately 2 weeks after spinal cord injury. Autonomic hyperreflexia is massive disinhibited reflex autonomic discharge in response to cutaneous or visceral stimulation below the level of the spinal cord lesion. It begins 1–3 weeks after spinal cord injury and the more distal the peripheral stimulation, the greater the sympathetic response. Therefore, the maximal sympathetic nervous system response results from stimulation of the ano-rectal area (S2–S4). The artery of Adamkiewicz arises from either an intercostal or lumbar branch of the aorta.

39. FFTFT

The normal forced expiratory volume in 1 second (FEV_1) is greater than 2–3 l. It is decreased in both asthma and emphysema. An FEV_1 of less than 70% predicted is associated with increased peri-operative morbidity. RV is normally 1–2 l and is increased in asthma and emphysema. Diffusion capacity is decreased in emphysema and is normal in asthmatics.

40. The larynx and its nerve supply
   A.   Sensory nerve supply is entirely derived from the vagus nerve
   B.   The right recurrent laryngeal nerve has a longer course than the left
   C.   Bilateral recurrent laryngeal nerve palsies lead to a hoarse voice
   D.   Cricothyroid muscle is supplied by the recurrent laryngeal nerve
   E.   The superior laryngeal nerve may be blocked percutaneously

41. Regarding hypothyroidism
   A.   Ninety per cent of patients are female
   B.   Patients have associated secondary hypercholesterolaemia
   C.   The full blood count may reveal a mild microcytic anaemia
   D.   The serum sodium may be low
   E.   The electrocardiograph may show bradycardia, high voltage changes and ischaemia

42. Hypomagnesaemia
   A.   Clinical features correlate with plasma levels
   B.   Is associated with diabetes mellitus
   C.   Causes vasospasm
   D.   Causes prolongation of the QT interval
   E.   Causes depressed tendon reflexes

40. TFFFT

The sensory nerve supply to the larynx is derived entirely from the vagus nerve. The left recurrent laryngeal nerve has a longer course than the right. Bilateral recurrent laryngeal nerve palsies lead to dyspnoea and inspiratory stridor with complete loss of vocal power. Cricothyroid is supplied by the superior laryngeal nerve. The superior laryngeal nerve may be blocked percutaneously by an injection placed inferior to the greater cornu of the hyoid bone.

41. TTFTF

The prevalence of hypothyroidism is 2/1000 women. Ninety per cent are women who can present at any age but are most commonly seen after middle age. Symptoms are non-specific at first. Secondary hypercholesterolaemia may be present at diagnosis and leads to accelerated atherosclerosis. A macrocytic anaemia may be present in hypothyroidism alone and a megaloblastic picture will suggest concomitant pernicious anaemia. Inappropriate ADH secretion can cause hyponatraemia. The ECG will show low voltage complexes.

42. FTTTF

As 1% of total body magnesium is extracellular, clinical features correlate poorly with plasma levels. Hypomagnesaemia is associated with poorly controlled diabetes mellitus. It causes both vasospasm and prolongation of the Q–T interval. Depressed tendon reflexes are a sign of hypermagnesaemia.

43. Concerning peri-operative cardiovascular monitoring
   A.   The CM5 configuration of ECG electrodes requires placement of the right arm electrode onto the manubrium and the left arm electrode in the V5 position
   B.   Blood pressure monitors which use the oscillometric method of blood pressure measurement (e.g. Dinamap) tend to underestimate the mean arterial blood pressure at low blood pressures, e.g. <80 mmHg
   C.   Parallel-sided Teflon cannulae reduce the incidence of radial artery thrombosis when used to measure intra-arterial blood pressure
   D.   When measuring indirect blood pressure, the cuff width should be 40–50% of the arm circumference
   E.   The activated clotting time (ACT) is linearly related to heparin dose up to an ACT value of 500–600 s

44. Concerning pulse oximetry
   A.   The two wavelengths of light emitted by a pulse oximeter are approximately 660 nm and 940 nm
   B.   Carboxyhaemoglobin has a similar absorbance to deoxyhaemoglobin at 660 nm, resulting in falsely low readings of oxygen saturation
   C.   Oxygen saturation readings can be inaccurate in neonates due to high concentrations of fetal haemoglobin
   D.   Inaccuracies can occur in patients with severe tricuspid regurgitation
   E.   Oxygen saturation readings are unaffected in the jaundiced patient

43. TFTFT

The CM5 configuration requires the ECG monitor to be set at lead 1 and is useful as a monitor of anterior ischaemia. Devices that use oscillometric methods to determine blood pressure tend to overestimate when the pressure is low. The cuff width should be 30–40% of the arm circumference.

44. TFFTT

In addition to knowing the wavelengths of light used by a pulse oximeter, it is useful for exam purposes to remember that the isobestic point for oxy- and deoxyhaemoglobin occurs at 805 nm. Carboxyhaemoglobin has a similar absorbance to oxyhaemoglobin at 660 nm, therefore giving a falsely high reading for oxygen saturation. Fetal haemoglobin has no major effect on pulse oximetry as it has a similar absorbance spectrum to haemoglobin A. Due to abnormally high venous pulsation in tricuspid regurgitation, the oximeter will measure venous, as well as arterial oxygen saturation. Methylene blue results in a severe decrease in measured oxygen saturation, as does blue nail polish with absorbance near 660 nm. Other nail polishes have a smaller effect while bilirubin has no effect.

45. Concerning nitrous oxide cylinders
- A. Nitrous oxide cylinders are made from an aluminium alloy
- B. The filling ratio is the weight of nitrous oxide in the cylinder divided by the weight of nitrous oxide it could hold when full
- C. The filling ratio for nitrous oxide in the UK is 0.7
- D. The pressure in a full nitrous oxide cylinder is 750 psi at 20°C
- E. The pressure gauge of a nitrous oxide cylinder only reflects the amount of vapour left in the cylinder once 90% of it has been used up

46. Regarding the side effects of non-steroidal anti-inflammatory drugs (NSAIDs)
- A. Gastropathy is due to a local irritant effect of NSAIDs on the gastric mucosa
- B. Platelet adhesion is reduced due to the irreversible inhibition of thromboxane A_2 in platelets
- C. Renal blood flow is reduced by NSAIDs due to a reduction in the prostaglandin-dependent portion of renal blood flow
- D. Renal impairment is more common than haematological side effects following the use of ketorolac
- E. Ketorolac is relatively contraindicated in asthmatic patients

47. The sitting position in neurosurgery is associated with
- A. Increased blood loss
- B. Quadriplegia
- C. Airway swelling
- D. Sciatic nerve damage
- E. Air embolism

45. FFFTF

Nitrous oxide cylinders, which have to withstand high pressures, are made from molybdenum steel, whereas an aluminium alloy is used to make cylinders which contain small quantities of gas at low pressure, e.g. cyclopropane. The pressure gauge of a nitrous oxide cylinder only reflects the amount of vapour left in the cylinder when 75% has been used up.

The filling ratio =

$$\frac{\text{Weight of gas in the cylinder}}{\text{Weight of water the cylinder could hold when full}}$$

The filling ratio for nitrous oxide in the UK is 0.75, whereas in tropical climates it is 0.65.

46. FTTFT

The gastropathy associated with NSAIDs occurs due to a reduction in the protective action on the gastric mucosa of prostaglandins. NSAIDs also reduce gastric mucosal blood flow and mucus production. Renal blood flow is particularly dependent on prostaglandins in the following patients: the elderly, patients with congestive cardiac failure, those undergoing major surgery, and those involved in trauma. NSAIDs reversibly reduce this portion of renal blood flow. The most common side effects associated with ketorolac, in descending order, are gastrointestinal, haematological and renal.

47. FTTTT

Blood loss is reduced in the sitting position due to increased venous drainage. Both quadriplegia and airway swelling have occurred secondary to extreme neck flexion. Sciatic nerve damage may arise secondary to stretching of the nerve. Air embolism is a particular risk due to the height of the cerebral veins above the heart.

48. Regarding obesity and body mass index (BMI)
   A.   BMI is defined as weight (kg)/height (m)^2
   B.   Desirable weight is a BMI of 5–10
   C.   Mild obesity is a BMI of 15–20
   D.   Moderate obesity is a BMI of 40–50
   E.   Severe obesity is a BMI >50

49. Amniotic fluid embolism is associated with
   A.   Raised pulmonary artery occlusion pressure
   B.   Right ventricular failure
   C.   Hypercoagulability
   D.   Convulsions
   E.   First trimester abortion

50. Regarding the measurement of temperature
   A.   The resistance of platinum increases with increasing temperature
   B.   A thermistor is a semiconductor
   C.   The fall in resistance of a thermistor with temperature is linear
   D.   The Seebeck effect describes the change in resistance of a metal oxide when it is heated
   E.   A thermocouple requires a battery to provide a current

48. TFFFF

You either know it or you don't. The degree of obesity is measured by skin-fold thickness but this is unreliable and BMI is the best index. The definition is correct and defines the limits of desirable weight (O), mild (I), moderate (II), and severe (III) for a given height. The boundaries are desirable (BMI 20–25), mild (BMI 25–30), moderate (BMI 30–40), and severe (BMI >40). It is a good idea to answer questions on obesity by defining it and then stating the causes: dietary, drugs, diseases.

49. TTTTT

Amniotic fluid embolism causes pulmonary vascular spasm which leads to raised pulmonary artery occlusion pressure and right ventricular failure. Disseminated intravascular coagulation follows a brief period of hypercoagulability. Convulsions may occur and result in cerebral insufficiency. Amniotic fluid embolism has been reported following first trimester abortion.

50. TTFFF

The resistance of metals increases and the current flow through them decreases with increasing temperature. Resistance thermometers usually use a platinum wire incorporated into a Wheatstone bridge circuit where the current flow through it from a battery is measured using a galvanometer. The resistance in a thermistor, which is a semiconductor, falls exponentially with increasing temperature. A thermocouple is produced at the junction of two different metal conductors where an electromotive force is set up (the Seebeck effect). The size of the voltage is dependent on the temperature difference between the two junctions. Therefore, if one junction is kept at a known reference temperature, the other reflects the temperature being measured.

51. **Regarding circle breathing systems and carbon dioxide absorption**
    A.   Barium lime is less efficient, weight for weight, than soda lime in the absorption of carbon dioxide
    B.   For the most efficient use of fresh gas flow, the unidirectional valves should be close to the patient
    C.   Barium lime is composed of 80% calcium hydroxide
    D.   Relative humidity can approach 100% using low flow rates
    E.   Ethyl violet is used as an indicator in soda lime and turns from violet to yellow when the soda lime is exhausted

52. **Concerning neuroaxial block**
    A.   Blood levels of local anaesthetic are highest following thoracic placement
    B.   Respiratory arrest following high blocks is due to phrenic nerve paralysis
    C.   The ligamentum flavum is narrowest in the thoracic region
    D.   High blocks are associated with a drop in expiratory reserve volume
    E.   The risk of dural tap is higher in the thoracic region than in the lumbar region

53. **Familial hypercholesterolaemia**
    A.   Is an autosomal-recessive condition
    B.   Is often race-specific
    C.   One in 500 of the population are heterozygotes
    D.   The genetic defect is at the high-density lipoprotein receptor
    E.   Tendon xanthomata occur

51. TTTTF

Barium lime is composed of 80% calcium hydroxide and 20% barium hydroxide which acts as a catalyst. Barium lime is 15% less efficient than soda lime in absorbing carbon dioxide. The size of the granules in both types of absorber is 4–8 mesh, i.e. 1/4–1/8 inch in the USA, and 3–10 mesh in the UK (this is favourite question!). Ethyl violet is added to both barium lime and soda lime. When pH decreases due to carbon dioxide absorption it changes from colourless to violet. Clayton yellow, another indicator, changes from deep pink when fresh, to off-white when exhausted.

52. FFFTT

Blood levels of local anaesthetic are highest following caudal anaesthesia due to the high vascularity of the caudal space. Following high blocks respiratory arrest is due to hypoperfusion of the respiratory centre secondary to profound hypotension. The ligamentum flavum is narrowest in the cervical region. High blocks are associated with a reduced expiratory reserve volume. The risk of dural tap is higher in the thoracic region than the lumbar region because of the reduced width of the epidural space.

53. FTTFT

Familial hypercholesterolaemia is an autosomal dominant condition and it is more common (up to 1/100 in some population groups) in Lebanese and South African Boers. The genetic defect is at the low density lipoprotein (LDL) receptor: LDL is inefficiently removed from the circulation and hence its half-life is prolonged. Patients have xanthomata which are cholesterol ester-laden foam cells. These are seen in tendons on the backs of the hand and on the tendon Achilles.

54. *Legionella pneumophila* pneumonia
A.   Is associated with a low-grade pyrexia
B.   Gastrointestinal symptoms are a feature
C.   Neurological signs are a feature
D.   Lymphocytosis is a feature
E.   Cefotaxime is currently the antibiotic of choice

55. Concerning the handling of drugs in patients with renal impairment
A.   Phenytoin is not effectively cleared from the plasma in patients receiving renal dialysis
B.   Most drug doses do not need to be modified until the glomerular filtration rate (GFR) has fallen to 25% of normal
C.   The action of suxamethonium is prolonged in patients with renal failure
D.   Procaine is contraindicated in renal failure as toxicity can occur due to reduced excretion
E.   The disposition of propofol is unaffected in patients with renal failure

56. Regarding humidification
A.   The Bernoulli effect is employed in the working of some humidifiers
B.   The unit of relative humidity is gH_2O/m^3
C.   The mass of water carried in saturated vapour is dependent on the temperature of the vapour
D.   The latent heat of vaporization of water is 2.43 MJ/kg
E.   The lower the environmental humidity in theatre the greater the risk of explosion due to static electricity

57. The following changes occur in the respiratory system of the obese
A.   Functional residual capacity drops
B.   Residual volume drops
C.   Expiratory reserve volume remains unchanged
D.   Thoracic compliance drops
E.   Total lung capacity remains unchanged

54. FTTFF

Presenting features of *Legionella pneumophila* pneumonia include a high fever, gastrointestinal and neurological symptoms. Lymphopenia is the norm. The antibiotic of choice is erythromycin.

55. TTFFT

Standard dialysis filters remove molecules whose molecular weight is less than 500. Drugs such as vancomycin are larger and are poorly cleared. Similarly, drugs which are extensively protein-bound, e.g. phenytoin, and drugs with a wide tissue distribution, e.g. digoxin, are poorly cleared by dialysis. If the GFR is greater than 30 ml/min, the doses of most drugs, except for some antibiotics and cardiac drugs, need not be reduced. Plasma cholinesterase is normal in patients with renal failure so that the actions and toxicity of suxamethonium and procaine, both of which are hydrolysed by plasma cholinesterase, are unaffected.

56. TFTTT

Nebulizers employ the Bernoulli effect in that a jet of air is used to entrain liquid from a reservoir, which then forms droplets. Absolute humidity is measured in grams per cubic metre (g/m^3) whereas relative humidity, the ratio between the absolute humidity and the humidity at saturation at the same temperature, is expressed as a percentage.

57. TFFTF

Owing to reduced thoracic compliance and the consequent increased work of breathing, functional residual capacity is reduced, primarily as a result of a reduced expiratory reserve volume. The residual volume remains unchanged. Total lung capacity decreases.

58. Regarding the local effects of pituitary tumours
  A.   Lateral extension leads to compression of the external ocular muscles
  B.   Downward extension into the sphenoid bone leads to cerebrospinal fluid rhinorrhoea
  C.   Upward extension leads to bitemporal hemianopia
  D.   In bitemporal hemianopia the lower temporal quadrant is affected first
  E.   Hypothalamic pressure does not lead to clinical symptoms

59. Regarding brainstem death testing
  A.   Two sets of tests must be performed at least 6 h apart
  B.   Testing must be delayed for 12 h following resumption of adequate circulation after a cardiac arrest
  C.   During the apnoea test the P_aCO_2 must rise above 6.65 kPa
  D.   The corneal reflex tests both the 5th and 7th cranial nerves
  E.   The testing is solely clinical in the UK

60. The partial pressure of oxygen
  A.   In the alveolus at sea level is 152 mmHg
  B.   Is equal to 21% of the atmospheric pressure at 30 000 feet
  C.   Depends on the temperature
  D.   In venous blood is 40 mmHg
  E.   In inspired gas is 101.3 kPa in a patient breathing 100% oxygen at sea level

58. TTTFF

Pressure can be directed towards the hypothalamus, laterally, downwards and upwards. Hypothalamic pressure causes the hypothalamic syndrome, which consists of polyphagia, altered temperature control, and thirst. Upwards extension leads to bi-temporal hemianopia and the upper temporal quadrants tend to be affected first. Larger tumours cause headaches, epilepsy, and symptoms of raised intracranial pressure. Downwards extension erodes the sphenoid bone causing cerebrospinal rhinorrhoea.

59. FFTTT

Two sets of tests must be performed; however, there is no minimum time limit between the two tests. Following a primary extracranial cause such as a cardiac arrest, 24 h must elapse following resumption of adequate circulation before the first set of tests can be performed. During the apnoea test P_aCO_2 must rise above 6.65 kPa. The corneal reflex has the 5th nerve as its afferent limb and the 7th nerve as its efferent limb. In the UK the tests are solely clinical in nature.

60. FTFTT

The partial pressure of oxygen in the atmosphere is approximately $20\% \times 760 = 152$ mmHg. In the alveolus the partial pressure of oxygen is $152 - 47 = 105$ mmHg where 47 mmHg is the partial pressure of water vapour in fully saturated alveolar gas at 37°C. Partial pressure is independent of temperature.

61. Local anaesthetics
   A. Raising the intracellular pH increases the speed of onset
   B. Local anaesthetics preferentially bind to the resting ion channel
   C. The maximum dose of plain bupivacaine is 2 mg/kg
   D. Bupivacaine cardiac toxicity is mediated by binding to fast sodium channels
   E. Optical isomers of bupivacaine differ in their anaesthetic potency

62. Hypokalaemia occurs in
   A. Cushing's syndrome
   B. Conn's syndrome
   C. Addison's disease
   D. Renal tubular acidosis
   E. Laxative administration

63. Meningitis in the adult population
   A. *Streptococcus pneumoniae* has the highest incidence
   B. *Haemophilus influenzae* has the poorest prognosis
   C. Ampicillin is the drug of choice for *Haemophilus influenzae* infection
   D. Lumbar puncture is the initial investigation of choice
   E. In bacterial meningitis, CSF glucose is raised

64. Effects of smoke inhalation include
   A. Deactivation of surfactant
   B. Decrease in alveolar surface tension
   C. Decreased pulmonary vascular resistance
   D. Pulmonary neutrophil recruitment
   E. Death commonly occurs due to ARDS

61. FFTTF

Raising the extracellular pH decreases onset time; however, changing the intracellular pH does not alter the onset time. Binding of local anaesthetics to ion channels occurs preferentially to activated channels rather than to resting ones. Bupivacaine cardiac toxicity is mediated by binding to fast sodium channels. L-bupivacaine dissociates more rapidly from this channel than the D-isomer, reducing the potential for cardiac toxicity.

62. TTFTT

The causes of hypokalaemia are three-fold: inadequate intake, gastrointestinal loss and renal loss. Gastrointestinal loss includes diarrhoea, villous adenoma and use of laxatives. Renal loss occurs in metabolic alkalosis (diuretics most commonly, liquorice, vomiting, and Barter's, Conn's and Cushing's syndromes), and metabolic acidosis (renal tubular acidosis, diabetic ketoacidosis and acetazolamide).

63. TFFFF

In the adult population *Streptococcus pneumoniae* has the highest incidence and is also associated with the worst prognosis. As there is an increasing incidence of ampicillin resistance in *Haemophilus influenzae*, cefotaxime is currently the antibiotic of choice. A CT scan should be performed prior to a lumbar puncture to exclude raised intracranial pressure. In bacterial meningitis CSF glucose levels are reduced.

64. TFFTF

Smoke inhalation deactivates surfactant resulting in an increased alveolar surface tension. Pulmonary vascular resistance increases. Neutrophils are recruited to the lungs in large quantities. Sepsis rather than ARDS is the common cause of death in this group of patients.

65. In measuring the concentration of volatile anaesthetic agents
   A.   The refractive index of light alters depending on the concentration of anaesthetic vapour being measured
   B.   The Riken gas analyser uses the principle that anaesthetic vapours absorb infrared light
   C.   The Raman scattering technique requires the use of an argon laser
   D.   Oxygen, nitrogen and carbon dioxide absorb infrared light
   E.   The Dräger Narkotest depends on the effect of volatile anaesthetics on silicone rubber

66. Functional residual capacity (FRC) is increased by
   A.   PEEP
   B.   Asthma
   C.   Reduced respiratory muscle tone
   D.   Pregnancy
   E.   Emphysema

67. Thyroid storm
   A.   Has an insidious onset
   B.   Most often occurs intra-operatively
   C.   May present with mental changes
   D.   Potassium iodide is not useful in the management
   E.   Steroids are useful in the management

65. TFTFT

The Riken gas indicator measures the difference between the refractive index of light in clean air and air containing another gas. Asymmetric polyatomic molecules absorb infrared light. Thus carbon dioxide, nitrous oxide, anaesthetic vapours and water vapour do, whereas oxygen and nitrogen do not absorb infrared light. When gas particles are bombarded with energy of a particular wavelength, they scatter energy at different wavelengths. The shift in wavelength is specific to each type of molecule. This is Raman scattering and an argon laser is the source of energy (wavelength 488 nm). The elasticity of rubber changes when anaesthetics dissolve in it.

66. TTFFT

FRC is increased by factors that reduce the tendency of the lung to recoil, e.g. asthma, emphysema and factors that increase the outward pull of the thoracic cage, e.g. PEEP. Upward displacement of the diaphragm, e.g. pregnancy and the supine position, and a reduction in respiratory muscle tone, e.g. general anaesthesia, reduce FRC.

67. FFTFT

Thyroid storm has an abrupt onset that most often occurs in the post-operative period. It has been known to present as mental changes such as mania or confusion. Both potassium iodide and steroids are useful in its treatment.

68. Malignant hyperthermia
  A. During a fulminating attack, minimal acid–base changes are a sinister sign
  B. Intracranial hypertension is a feature
  C. Insulin and glucose are the optimal method of controlling hyperkalaemia
  D. Incidence is increased in anxious patients
  E. Active cooling should be terminated at 37°C

69. Regarding the anaemia of chronic renal failure
  A. Decreased erythropoietin production is the major cause of the anaemia
  B. The severity of the anaemia correlates with the decrease in glomerular filtration rate
  C. Haemoglobin levels drop within a few days of the onset of acute renal failure
  D. A side effect of erythropoietin administration is exacerbation of hypertension
  E. Aluminium intoxication is a cause of anaemia in renal failure

70. Paediatric trauma
  A. Spinal cord trauma is rare in children
  B. Cervical spinal cord trauma most commonly occurs in the mid-to-low regions
  C. Spinal cord trauma in the absence of a radiologically visible lesion is rare
  D. Children are as likely as adults to have an intracranial lesion
  E. Seizures occur with similar incidence to adult trauma

71. Regarding endocrine glands
  A. The hypothalamus secretes dopamine
  B. The anterior pituitary gland secretes anti-diuretic hormone
  C. The posterior pituitary gland secretes prolactin
  D. The adrenal cortex secretes cortisone
  E. The testes secret inhibin

68. TTFTF

During a fulminating attack of malignant hyperthermia minimal acid–base changes indicate a falling cardiac output and death rapidly ensues. Intracranial hypertension arises secondary to hypoxia and acidosis. The optimal method of controlling hyperkalaemia is termination of the malignant hyperthermia by administration of dantrolene. Very rarely malignant hyperthermia has been induced in the absence of triggering agents, anxiety reactions precipitating an apparent malignant hyperthermia response. Active cooling methods should be stopped at 38–39°C to avoid excessive cooling.

69. TTTTT

Many factors contribute to the anaemia of renal disease. Deficiency states (iron, folate, B_{12}), endocrine dysfunction (decreased erythropoietin production being the most important), direct effects of uraemia, exogenous toxins, and increased catabolism (intercurrent infection) all contribute. Erythropoietin administration is very effective in raising haemoglobin levels but it exacerbates or causes hypertension.

70. TFFFF

Spinal cord trauma in children accounts for 5% of the total incidence of this form of trauma. In the first decade cervical spine trauma occurs almost exclusively in the first two spinal segments. In 50% of cases spinal cord trauma occurs in the absence of a radiologically visible injury. In children trauma less commonly results in an intracranial collection than adults, but seizures as a consequence of trauma occur more commonly than in adults.

71. TFFFT

It is important not to forget basic physiological knowledge for this examination. The adrenal cortex secretes cortisol!

72. Concerning haemoglobin
   A.   Methaemoglobin and carboxyhaemoglobin shift the
         oxygen dissociation curve to the left ˙
   B.   Acute intermittent porphyria (AIP) occurs due to
         increased production of the porphyrin precursors
         amino-laevulinic acid and porphobilinogen in the red
         blood cell
   C.   Ketamine induces porphyria and is unsafe for use in
         porphyric patients
   D.   β-thalassaemia is associated with abnormal
         haemoglobins including HbS and HbC
   E.   Following acute blood loss, erythropoietin
         concentration increases within 6 h

73. Regarding ventilation using a T-piece
   A.   To avoid rebreathing, the recommended fresh gas flow
         rate in a spontaneously breathing 15 kg child is
         7.5 l/min
   B.   During controlled ventilation in children using a
         Mapleson F system, fresh gas flow rates (litres per
         minute) should be 1000 ml/min + 100 ml/kg/min to
         avoid rebreathing
   C.   The Bain system was described in 1972
   D.   The outer tube of a Bain circuit is 25 mm in diameter
         and 1.8 m long
   E.   Trunk ventilation can be used with the Bain circuit for
         controlled ventilation

74. Dantrolene
   A.   At doses of 10 mg/kg paralysis ensues
   B.   May be dissolved in 5% dextrose
   C.   Requires sodium hydroxide to dissolve
   D.   Should be administered pre-operatively to
         MH-susceptible patients
   E.   Increases sarcoplasmic reuptake of calcium

72. TFFTT

Methaemoglobin contains iron in the oxidized ferric (Fe^{3+}) form, while carboxyhaemoglobin contains carbon monoxide which has 250 times more affinity for haemoglobin than oxygen. In both cases, this results in a decrease in oxygen-carrying capacity and a compensatory increase in the affinity of the remaining normal haemoglobin for oxygen. This shifts the oxygen dissociation curve to the left, further impairing peripheral oxygen delivery. AIP is due to abnormal synthesis of porphyrin in the liver. Unsafe drugs in porphyric patients include barbiturates, etomidate, diazepam, steroids, pancuronium and phenytoin.

73. TTTFT

To avoid rebreathing using a T-piece in a spontaneously breathing patient, the fresh gas flow rate should be $3 \times (1000\,\text{ml/min} + 100\,\text{ml/kg/min})$ which is 7.5 l/min for a 15 kg child. During controlled ventilation in children, although the fresh gas flow rate is $1000 + 100\,\text{ml/kg/min}$, the minimum should be 3 l/min to maintain normocapnia. Bain and Spoerel described the Bain system in 1972. It is a coaxial Mapleson system that is 1.8 m long with an outer tube diameter of 22 mm.

74. FFTFF

At maximum doses dantrolene produces a mild muscle weakness preserving the ability to cough and take a deep breath. Dantrolene should not be dissolved in crystalloid solutions as they decrease its solubility. Dantrolene requires a high pH to dissolve, which is why sodium hydroxide is used. Pre-operative dantrolene is no longer administered as anaesthesia without triggering agents is almost always uneventful. Dantrolene reduces sarcoplasmic release of calcium without altering its re-uptake.

75. Low-molecular-weight heparin
- A. Peak anticoagulant effect occurs 1–2 h following subcutaneous injection
- B. Metabolism is via a similar pathway to standard heparin
- C. Protamine fully reverses the anticoagulant effect
- D. There should be a 6 h delay from the last subcutaneous dose prior to siting a neuroaxial block
- E. Anticoagulant activity is as predictable as that of standard heparin

76. The features of the peripheral neuropathy of diabetes mellitus are
- A. Rapid onset
- B. Asymmetrical distribution
- C. Wasting, particularly of the hands and feet
- D. Loss of vibration sense is an early sign
- E. Hypoaesthesia and dysaesthesia are usually confined to the hands

77. Necrotizing fasciitis
- A. Type I infections are caused by group A streptococci
- B. There is often a preceding history of minor trauma
- C. Late lesions may be pain-free
- D. Treatment with antibiotics alone is usually successful
- E. Hyperbaric oxygen is beneficial

75. FFFFF

Following a subcutaneous injection of low molecular weight heparin (LMWH) peak anticoagulant effects occur at 3–4 h. LMWH is almost solely renally excreted whereas standard heparin is metabolized after binding to endothelial cells and macrophages. Unlike standard heparin, LMWH is only partially reversed by protamine. Owing to the prolonged activity of LMWH there should be a delay of 8–12 h prior to siting a neuroaxial block. The anticoagulant effect of LMWH is more predictable than that of standard heparin.

76. FFTTF

The peripheral neuropathy of diabetes mellitus is characterized by the following features: insidious onset, symmetrical distribution, reduced or painful sensation confined to the feet and legs, an early loss of vibration sense, motor involvement which is evident as wasting of the small muscles of the hands and feet, and accompanying reflex abnormalities (absent ankle jerks). Other diabetic neuropathies include the mononeuropathies of the peripheral nerves (lateral cutaneous nerve of the thigh, ulnar and median nerves, and the cranial nerves I, IV, and VI) and, of course, an autonomic neuropathy.

77. FTTFF

Type I necrotizing fasciitis is usually caused by enteric bowel organisms or vibrio species. Type II is caused by group A streptococci. A history of preceding minor trauma is common. Owing to necrosis of nerve fibres late lesions are often pain free. Successful treatment involves both antibiotics and extensive surgical debridement. Hyperbaric oxygen is not beneficial.

78. **The following substances are renal arteriolar dilators**
    A. PGE_2
    B. Adrenaline
    C. Thromboxane A_2
    D. ANP
    E. Dopamine

79. **The electrocardiographic changes of hyperkalaemia include**
    A. Peaked T waves
    B. Peaked R waves
    C. Peaked P waves
    D. Shortened PR interval
    E. Sine waves

80. **The following are gases at room temperature**
    A. Entonox
    B. Air
    C. Oxygen/helium mixture
    D. Nitrogen
    E. Xenon

81. **Regarding the storage and delivery of pipeline anaesthetic gases**
    A. The temperature of oxygen inside a vacuum-insulated evaporator (VIE) is approximately $-175°C$
    B. Oxygen concentrators use a zeolite that absorbs nitrogen, producing 92% oxygen from air
    C. The gas produced by oxygen concentrators contains 5% argon which can cause pulmonary vascular damage if breathed for long periods of time
    D. All pipeline gases reaching theatre contain gas at a pressure of approximately 4 bar
    E. The British standard for a medical vacuum system requires a vacuum of 533 mbar below atmospheric pressure and an air flow of at least 60 l/min to be maintained at each outlet

78. TFFFT

ANP dilates the afferent arteriole while constricting the efferent arteriole. As α receptors are in greater number in the renal arterioles than β receptors, adrenaline has a constrictor effect. PGE_2 and dopamine both cause renal arteriolar dilatation. Thromboxane A_2 causes renal arteriolar vasoconstriction.

79. TFFFT

The electrocardiographic changes of hyperkalaemia occur in the following sequence: peaked T waves, diminished R waves, widening of the QRS complex, prolonged PR interval, loss of the P wave, and finally sine waves. The plasma level of potassium is no indicator of a patient's response to the hyperkalaemia.

80. TTTTT

A gas cannot be compressed into a liquid whatever the pressure applied to it. A substance is a gas at the temperature concerned if this temperature is above the critical temperature of that substance. Vapours, on the other hand, can be compressed into a liquid. At room temperature therefore, nitrous oxide, carbon dioxide and cyclopropane are vapours.

81. TTFFF

Zeolites are hydrated aluminium silicates of the alkaline earth metals that preferentially adsorb nitrogen from air passed over them. Five per cent argon can be produced by oxygen concentrators although the concentration is usually much less (0.9%). Argon has no adverse effects. Most piped gases to theatre are at a pressure of 4 bar. The exception is air. There are two air pipelines, one for medical purposes at a pressure of 4 bar, and one to drive power tools, e.g. saws, at 7 bar. For medical vacuum, although the pressure should be 533 mbar below atmospheric, the flow rate need only be 40 l/min and not 60 l/min.

82. Coarctation of the aorta is associated with
  A.   An equal male:female sex incidence
  B.   Klinefelter's syndrome
  C.   A mid-systolic murmur
  D.   Notching of the upper anterior ribs
  E.   Mitral valve abnormalities

83. The causes of respiratory alkalosis include
  A.   Asthma
  B.   Emphysema
  C.   Pulmonary embolism
  D.   Midbrain lesion
  E.   Barbiturate poisoning

84. Regarding pulmonary hypertension
  A.   It is defined as a mean pulmonary arterial pressure of >30 mmHg at rest
  B.   It is defined as a mean pulmonary arterial pressure of >30 mmHg on exercise
  C.   Primary pulmonary hypertension is the most common cause
  D.   Anticoagulant therapy should be given to all patients with secondary pulmonary hypertension
  E.   Advanced disease causes tricuspid regurgitation and massive 'c' waves in the jugular venous wave

82. FFTFT

Coarctation of the aorta affects males more than females in a ratio of 2:1. It is associated with Turner's syndrome. The murmur of coarctation of the aorta is usually mid-systolic. However, if severe, with a well developed collateral circulation, the murmur is continuous. Characteristic rib notching of the inferior borders of posterior ribs 4–9 is due to erosion by dilated and tortuous intercostal arteries. The associated cardiac abnormalities include patent ductus arteriosus, bicuspid aortic valve, ventriculoseptal defect and mitral valve abnormalities.

83. TTTTF

This is straightforward. The causes of a respiratory alkalosis are respiratory disease (asthma, pneumonia, emboli), central nervous system causes (psychogenic or midbrain lesions), general causes (early shock, fever), metabolic (drugs – aspirin poisoning, liver disease) and pregnancy.

84. FTFFF

The definition is a mean pulmonary arterial pressure greater than 20 mmHg at rest and at least 30 mmHg on exercise with a normal pulmonary occlusion pressure. Primary pulmonary hypertension is rare and is more common in relatively young women. The secondary causes are left-sided heart disease, thromboembolism, chronic lung disease, congenital cardiac disease with left-to-right shunts, and peripheral pulmonary artery stenoses. Advanced disease causes systolic 'v' waves in the jugular venous waveform. The patients present with exertional dyspnoea, chest pain, syncope, and rarely sudden death.

85. Hypothermia is associated with
A. Hypotonia
B. Absent pupillary reflexes
C. Reduced stroke volume
D. Atrial flutter
E. Prolonged PR interval

86. The following therapies are useful in the management of phantom limb pain
A. TENS
B. Opioids
C. Carbamazepine
D. Ketamine
E. Tricyclic antidepressants

87. The following statements are true
A. Atropine is more effective than glycopyrrolate at inhibiting the gastrointestinal effects of neostigmine on reversal of neuromuscular blockade
B. The MAC of inhalational anaesthetics falls linearly with the temperature of the patient
C. The magnetic field set up by an MRI scanner is less than the Earth's magnetic field
D. In patients with hepatic cirrhosis, a grade D Child and Turcotte classification carries a worse prognosis than a grade A
E. The incidence of adverse hypersensitivity reaction to hydroxyethyl starch is greater than that to dextrans

88. The following statements regarding drug interactions with neuromuscular blocking agents (NMBA) are true
A. Aminoglycosides potentiate competitive NMBA
B. Lithium potentiates the effect of competitive NMBA
C. Magnesium potentiates the effect of competitive NMBA
D. Ecothiopate eye drops potentiate the effects of mivacurium
E. High-dose digoxin has been shown to block the effects of suxamethonium in vitro

85. FTFTT

As hypothermia progresses the patient becomes hypertonic and at temperatures below 27°C the pupillary response to light is lost. Cardiac output falls due to a reduction in rate, while stroke volume is maintained. Hypothermia is associated with atrial flutter and an increased PR interval.

86. TFTTF

TENS, carbamazepine and ketamine have been shown to be useful. Phantom limb pain does not respond to opioids, and tricyclic antidepressants are of no proven benefit.

87. TTFFT

The fall in MAC with temperature is related to the change in lipid solubility of the agent with temperature. The MAC of halothane falls by 5% per degree Celsius. A 2 tesla magnetic field is set up by an MRI scanner compared to the Earth's magnetic field of 0.00005 tesla. The mortality associated with the Child and Turcotte classification of liver disease is: A 5%, B 10%, C >50%. There is no class D (sorry!). Included in the classification are serum bilirubin, serum albumin, ascites, encephalopathy and nutritional state. There are 1 in 1200 allergic reactions to hydroxyethyl starch compared to 1 in 3000 with dextrans.

88. TTTTF

Aminoglycosides reduce the presynaptic release of acetylcholine, while at high doses they also act postsynaptically. Hypermagnesaemia potentiates neuromuscular blockade by decreasing acetylcholine release and reducing the sensitivity of the muscle end-plate to acetylcholine. Ecothiopate eye drops inhibit plasma cholinesterase, potentiating the effect of both mivacurium and suxamethonium. Suxamethonium enhances digoxin toxicity.

89. Regarding hepatitis C
- A.   It accounts for nearly all cases of post-transfusion hepatitis
- B.   Subtype Ib appears the least virulent
- C.   It commonly causes acute hepatitis
- D.   It commonly causes fulminant hepatic failure
- E.   Most patients become chronic carriers and develop cirrhosis

90. The following are adverse effects of drugs used to treat rheumatoid arthritis
- A.   Nephrotoxicity is more common in patients treated with penicillamine than in those treated with gold
- B.   Penicillamine is associated with a positive Coombs' test
- C.   Aspirin may increase the risk of methotrexate toxicity
- D.   Gold causes a membranous glomerular nephropathy, leading to the nephrotic syndrome
- E.   Cyclosporins potentiate the effect of competitive neuromuscular blocking agents

89. TFFFT

Hepatitis C is the main agent identified in post-transfusion hepatitis. There are several subtypes (I, II, III) and type Ib is the most virulent. Acute hepatitis rarely occurs and it more commonly causes chronic cryptogenic cirrhosis. It rarely, if ever, causes fulminant hepatic failure. Interferon-α may be of some benefit but there is no standard treatment.

90. FFTTF

Nephrotoxicity occurs in 4% of patients treated with penicillamine and 40% of those treated with gold. Penicillamine causes leucopenia, eosinophilia and thrombocytopenia but not a positive Coombs' test. Rarely it causes a myasthenia-like autoimmune reaction. Methotrexate causes GI upset, bone marrow toxicity, renal failure and interstitial lung and alveolar fibrosis. NSAIDs may increase the risk of toxicity by displacing methotrexate from plasma proteins and reducing renal excretion of the drug. Cyclosporins are nephrotoxic.

Paper 5

1. **Concerning medical cylinders**
    A. Size H is the largest cylinder
    B. Size E cylinders contain 680 l of oxygen
    C. The pin index configuration for nitrous oxide is 2 and 5
    D. The pressure in a full entonox cylinder is the same as the pressure in a full oxygen cylinder
    E. Helium is presented in brown cylinders with brown-and-white quartered shoulders

2. **Regarding heparin**
    A. Heparin inhibits the action of antithrombin III
    B. Heparin increases blood vessel wall permeability
    C. The side effect of thrombocytopenia is equally common following either porcine or bovine heparin
    D. 1 mg of protamine sulphate reverses the effect of 100 units of heparin
    E. Low-molecular-weight heparin contains the fraction of heparin with a molecular weight $<7\,kDa$

1. FTFTF

The sizes of medical cylinders are as follows:

B	330×76 mm
C	430×89 mm
D	535×102 mm
E	865×102 mm
F	930×140 mm
AF	670×175 mm
G	1320×178 mm
J	1520×229 mm.

The pin index system was designed to prevent cylinders of different gases from being interchangeable. The pin index configuration for nitrous oxide is the 3 and 5 position, while 2 and 5 is the configuration for oxygen cylinders. The pressure inside both full entonox and oxygen cylinders at 15°C is 137×100 kPa. The pressure inside a full nitrous oxide cylinder is 44×100 kPa. Helium is contained in brown cylinders with brown shoulders while heliox (79% He/21% O_2) is stored in brown cylinders with brown and white quartered shoulders.

2. FTFTT

Heparin is a co-factor for antithrombin III and enhances its ability to inactivate thrombin and the activated factors IX, X, XI, XII. It also inhibits platelet function and increases the permeability of blood vessels. At doses producing an equivalent antithrombotic effect, low molecular weight heparin (below 7 kDa) causes fewer complications. It works predominantly by catalysing the inhibition of factor Xa by antithrombin III, with little activity against thrombin. Low molecular weight heparins have relatively long half-lives and can be given once daily. Thrombocytopenia, which has an immunological aetiology, is more common following bovine than porcine heparin. Osteoporosis can occur following long-term heparin therapy.

3. Sevoflurane
A. Has a chiral centre
B. Contains chlorine groups
C. Is 3–5% metabolized
D. Has a vapour pressure of 243 mmHg
E. Has a MAC of two in oxygen

4. Regarding myxoedema coma
A. It is precipitated by heat exposure
B. It is precipitated by barbiturates
C. It is a rare cause of hypernatraemia
D. It can lead to hyperglycaemia
E. It can be precipitated by intercurrent infections

5. The haemolytic uraemic syndrome
A. Is an uncommon cause of acute renal failure in childhood
B. The predominant age group is 4–6 years
C. Is mediated by an exotoxin
D. Both haemolysis and thrombocytopenia may arise
E. Fresh frozen plasma has been shown to be beneficial

6. Cerebral vasospasm
A. May be diagnosed by angiography, Doppler, somatosensory evoked potentials and direct visualization
B. In the affected region, $CMRO_2$ decreases
C. Treatment includes IV nimodipine
D. Transluminal balloon angioplasty may be performed prior to clipping the aneurysm
E. Hyponatraemia, but not hypernatraemia, may occur

3. **FFTFT**

   Sevoflurane does not have a chiral centre. It is halogenated by fluorine groups only. It is 3–5% metabolized. The vapour pressure of sevoflurane is 160 mmHg. It has a MAC of 2 in oxygen.

4. **FTFFT**

   Myxoedema coma is a rare medical emergency which presents mainly in elderly women. It is precipitated by cold exposure, intercurrent infections, barbiturates and phenothiazines. The patient presents with the features of hypothyroidism, coma and is often hypoglycaemic, and hyponatraemic. Treatment is by gradual warming, thyroxine 500 mcg intravenously, and treatment of electrolytic disorders. The prognosis is generally poor.

5. **FFFTF**

   The haemolytic uraemic syndrome is one of the most common causes of acute renal failure in children. The predominant age group is 6 months to 4 years. It is caused by endotoxin released by *E. coli* 0157. Both thrombocytopenia and haemolysis can occur. Fresh frozen plasma has not been shown to be of therapeutic benefit.

6. **TFTFF**

   Vasospasm may be diagnosed angiographically, by Doppler, by somatosensory evoked potentials and by direct vision during surgery. In the affected region, $CMRO_2$ remains unchanged. Treatment for vasospasm is oral, IV or NG nimodipine. Transluminal balloon angioplasty should not be performed in the presence of an unclipped aneurysm. Both hyper- and hyponatraemia can occur.

7. Cardiac contusions
   A. Occur in up to 30% of chest injuries
   B. Sinus tachycardia may be the only feature
   C. Elevations in serum creatinine kinase aid diagnosis
   D. Tricuspid valve damage rarely occurs
   E. Cardiac arrest may ensue

8. The following statements regarding osmosis are true
   A. 1 mmol of a salt which completely dissociates into two ions in solution provides 1 mosmole
   B. The osmotic pressure of a solution is proportional to the molecular weight of the substance dissolved in solution
   C. The main contribution to the osmotic pressure exerted by plasma comes from plasma proteins
   D. The osmolality of plasma is 280–305 mosmol/l
   E. Osmolality can be determined using a flame photometer

9. Local anaesthetic toxicity
   A. May lead to asystole
   B. Bupivacaine cardiac toxicity may have a central element
   C. Bupivacaine may cause cardiotoxic effects in the absence of CNS effects
   D. The refractory period of the cardiac action potential is increased
   E. Local anaesthetics exhibit a negative inotropic effect

7. **FTFTT**

   Cardiac contusions occur in up to 17% of blunt chest injuries. They may present with a number of ECG changes including a sinus tachycardia. Creatinine kinase is not a specific marker of myocardial damage in the presence of blunt trauma. The tricuspid valve is rarely involved to any significant degree. A complication of cardiac contusions includes cardiac arrest.

8. **FFFFT**

   The osmol is dependent on the number of completely dissociated ions of a salt in solution so that if 1 mmol of a salt dissociates into 2 ions in solution it provides 2 mosmol. Osmolarity is the number of osmols per litre (mosmol/l) of solution while osmolality is the number of osmols per kg (mosmol/kg) of solvent. Therefore the osmolality of plasma is 280–305 mosmol/kg. Sodium and its anions, urea and glucose are the greatest contributors to the osmolarity of plasma. Osmotic pressure is the pressure required to stop the passage of solvent in a solution by osmosis across a semipermeable membrane and is proportional to the number of particles per unit volume. The osmotic pressure of plasma is 7.3 atmospheres.

9. **TTTFT**

   Extremely high concentrations of local anaesthetics will prolong conduction time and lead to bradycardias and sinus arrest. The injection of bupivacaine into the brains of experimental animals has been shown to be arrhymogenic, which may indicate a central role in cardiac toxicity. Bupivacaine has also been shown to be arrhymogenic in the absence of CNS effects. Local anaesthetic toxicity reduces the cardiac action potential and the refractory period.

10. Regarding primary glomerulonephritis
  A. It accounts for 75% of patients with end-stage renal failure
  B. Captopril (>150 mg/day) can cause glomerulonephritis
  C. In the majority of cases the antigen is unknown
  D. In Berger's disease, urine complexes containing IgA are deposited in the mesangium
  E. Primary glomerulonephritis is defined as glomerular inflammation in which the kidneys are primarily affected, usually symmetrically

11. HIV-associated disease
  A. *Cryptococcus neoformans* meningitis presents with severe neck stiffness
  B. CMV most commonly affects the gut
  C. *Toxoplasma gondii* infection is ruled out by the absence of a positive antibody test
  D. A raised lactate dehydrogenase supports the diagnosis of *Pneumocystis carinii* pneumonia
  E. The majority of lymphomas are of the T-cell type

12. When feeding patients on the ITU
  A. The EMG is useful in assessing malnutrition
  B. Serum albumin is useful in assessing malnutrition
  C. Excessive glucose administration can lead to hypophosphataemia
  D. The Harris–Benedict equation calculates basal energy expenditure
  E. In sepsis, energy requirements may rise to 20 kcal/kg/day

10. FTTTT

If the kidneys are involved as part of a systemic disease the glomerulonephritis is known as secondary. Glomerulonephritis accounts for about 30% of patients with chronic renal failure. The majority of antigens are unknown. Known antigens are endogenous or exogenous. Endogenous antigens include neoplasia (lymphoma, leukaemia and carcinoma), DNA (SLE), immunoglobulin, and thyroglobulin. Exogenous antigens include viruses (hepatitis B and C), bacteria, parasites, drugs (captopril is the most likely one to be encountered by anaesthetists) and horse proteins.

11. FFTTF

Cryptococcus neoformans causes a meningitis in AIDS patients. Typically neck stiffness is mild or absent. CMV most commonly affects the retina. *Toxoplasma gondii* infection may be ruled out in the presence of a negative antibody test. The majority of lymphomas are of the B-cell type.

12. TFTTF

Muscle fatigue, detectable using the EMG, is consistently present in malnutrition. Serum albumin levels are not useful in the assessment of malnutrition. Hypophosphataemia is a recognized consequence of excessive glucose administration. The Harris–Benedict equation calculates basal energy expenditure. 20 kcal/kg/24h does not represent an increase in energy requirements.

13. Regarding Guillain–Barré syndrome

A. It typically begins a few weeks after an acute respiratory infection
B. Distal motor weakness occurs first
C. Motor symptoms affect the arms first and then 'descend'
D. It can occur at any stage of HIV infection
E. Cerebrospinal fluid analysis typically shows a low protein level with a lymphocytosis

14. The following are indications for haemofiltration on the ITU

A. Amitriptyline poisoning
B. Digoxin poisoning
C. Hyperthermia
D. Urea >40 mmol/l
E. Severe hyperkalaemia

15. Regarding the screening of relatives of patients with malignant hyperpyrexia (MH)

A. Blood levels of pyrophosphate are raised in nearly all MH-susceptible patients
B. During screening, the muscle strip being tested is prepared in dextrose saline
C. During screening, halothane and caffeine are applied separately to the muscle strip
D. The patient has MH syndrome (MHS) if a muscle strip taken from that patient contracts in response to either caffeine or halothane
E. Patients can be classified as either MH syndrome (MHS) or normal (MHN)

13. **FFFTF**
Guillain–Barré normally begins a few days after an acute infection. This is usually respiratory in nature. Distal paraesthesia occurs first and is normally followed by motor symptoms. The motor symptoms 'ascend'. Neurophysiological tests confirm the diagnosis – nerve conduction velocity is slowed but often only the proximal velocity is reduced. CSF shows an elevated CSF protein, but no CSF lymphocytosis. The presence of white cells should cause consideration of other diagnoses including HIV infection.

14. **FTTTT**
Amitriptyline is not effectively removed by haemofiltration. Digoxin clearance is enhanced by haemofiltration. Extracorporeal cooling methods may be employed in cases of refractory hyperthermia. Both uraemia and hyperkalaemia are indications for haemofiltration.

15. **FFTFF**
There is no reliable blood test to detect MH in patients. The muscle strip is prepared in Ringer's lactate solution. In Europe, halothane and caffeine are applied separately to the muscle strip to be tested. If the muscle contracts in the presence of both halothane and caffeine the patient is classified as having MH syndrome (MHS); however, if it contracts to only one substance the patient is MH equivocal (MHE), and if no contraction takes place at all the patient is MH normal (MHN).

16. **Concerning the use of infrared analysers to monitor gases and vapours**
    A. Carbon dioxide absorbs infrared light with a wavelength of $4.28\,\mu m$
    B. The Hook and Tucker meter uses the principle of infrared absorption by halothane
    C. The absorption band of infrared light by oxygen overlaps that of nitrous oxide
    D. Nitrogen does not absorb infrared light
    E. Nitrous oxide maximally absorbs infrared light at a wavelength of 200 nm

17. **The thromboelastograph may detect the following conditions**
    A. Fibrinolysis
    B. Haemophilia
    C. Hypercoagulability
    D. Aspirin-induced platelet dysfunction
    E. Heparin therapy

18. **Regarding diabetes mellitus**
    A. Insulin is a polypeptide composed of A and B chains
    B. Human proinsulin is a single polypeptide chain
    C. Proinsulin is broken down by proteolysis to insulin and C-peptide
    D. Hypoglycaemia decreases growth hormone
    E. Biguanides act by increasing the secretion of insulin by the pancreas

19. **Regarding croup**
    A. It is commonly caused by the parainfluenza type 1 virus
    B. It has a peak incidence at 6 years of age
    C. Oral paracetamol is contraindicated
    D. Nebulized adrenaline acts by stimulating α receptors in the subglottic mucosa
    E. Nebulized budesonide improves symptoms for the first 4 h after administration

16. TFFTF

Gases that have two or more different atoms in the molecule absorb infrared light. The Hook and Tucker halothane meter uses the principle of ultraviolet absorption to measure halothane concentration although anaesthetic vapours also absorb infrared light. Nitrous oxide absorbs infrared light with a wavelength of approximately 4.4 μm. Light with a wavelength of 200 nm is in the ultraviolet spectrum and is absorbed by halothane.

17. TTTFT

The thromboelastograph is unable to detect subtle abnormalities such as aspirin-induced platelet abnormalities.

18. TTTFF

The A chain has 21 aminoacids and the B chain 33. When produced normally by the pancreas, it is first manufactured as a larger molecule, proinsulin (a single polypeptide chain of 86 amino acids), from which a connecting fragment called C-peptide is split off leaving insulin. Different animal species have slight differences in the structure of insulin. Hypoglycaemia raises growth hormone levels and sulphonylureas are claimed to act by stimulating the islet cells to produce insulin.

19. TFFTT

Croup (laryngotracheobronchitis) has a peak incidence in the second year of life. Treatment consists of paracetamol to reduce the fever, and humidification. Whether humidification improves outcome or hastens recovery is unclear. Remember that the differential diagnosis includes bacterial epiglottitis, inhaled foreign body, bacterial tracheitis, paratonsillar abscess and angio-oedema. Nebulized adrenaline results in reduced swelling and oedema. Systemic corticosteroids have been shown to reduce the need for intubation.

20. The anatomy of the nose
   A. The middle turbinate is the largest
   B. The nasolacrimal duct enters the nasal cavity inferior to
       the middle turbinate
   C. The floor of the nasal cavity is innervated by the long
       sphenopalatine nerve
   D. The maxillary sinus drains into the middle meatus
   E. The nasal septum is innervated exclusively by branches
       of the maxillary nerve

**21. The following statements regarding the effects of alcohol on
     drug metabolism are true**
   A. The metabolism of warfarin is increased
   B. The metabolism of thiopentone is increased
   C. The metabolism of phenytoin is reduced
   D. The metabolism of aminophylline is unchanged
   E. The metabolism of local anaesthetics is delayed

22. Etomidate
   A. Is emetogenic
   B. Is an imidazole derivative
   C. Inhibits 17-α hydroxylase
   D. Injection is pain-free
   E. Inhibits sympathetic outflow

**23. The following are included in Child's classification of liver
     failure**
   A. Plasma bilirubin concentration
   B. Plasma albumin concentration
   C. Plasma alanine transferase (ALT) concentration
   D. Prothrombin time
   E. Severity of encephalopathy

20. FFFTF
The inferior turbinate is the largest. The nasolacrimal duct drains into the nasal cavity below the inferior turbinate. The floor of the nasal cavity is innervated anteriorly by the anterior superior dental nerve and posteriorly by the greater palatine nerve. The maxillary sinus drains into the middle meatus via the hiatus semilunaris. The anterior part of the nasal septum is suppled by branches of the ophthalmic nerve, the posterior part is supplied by branches of the maxillary nerve.

21. TTFTF
Alcohol is a liver enzyme inducer. It increases the metabolism of warfarin, barbiturates and phenytoin.

22. TTTFF
Etomidate is associated with a high incidence of post-operative nausea and vomiting. Etomidate predominantly inhibits 11-β hydroxylase and to a lesser extent 17-α hydroxylase. Pain on injection is a consistent feature of etomidate administration. Etomidate maintains cardiovascular stability by not attenuating sympathetic outflow.

23. TTFFT
As well as the factors mentioned in the question, Child's classification of liver failure includes the degree of ascites and the state of nutrition of the patient. The Pugh modification of Child's classification replaces nutritional state with prothrombin time.

24. The ulnar nerve
    A.   Is derived from C7, C8 and T1
    B.   Is formed lateral to the axillary artery
    C.   Supplies the medial head of triceps
    D.   Lies deep to the flexor retinaculum
    E.   Lies lateral to the head of flexor carpi ulnaris

25. Regarding hepatitis B
    A.   About 50% of patients become chronic carriers
    B.   Twenty per cent of chronic carriers develop cirrhosis and hepatic cellular carcinoma
    C.   Babies born to mothers who are chronic carriers or who have hepatitis B should be given immunoglobulin at birth and be vaccinated
    D.   Vaccination titres of anti-HbS >100 IU/ml imply good immunity
    E.   Hepatitis B rarely resolves completely

26. Risk factors for the development of nosocomial pulmonary infection in the ITU are
    A.   Endotracheal intubation
    B.   The presence of a nasogastric tube
    C.   Length of stay
    D.   Intravenous H_2 antagonist therapy
    E.   Male gender

27. Secondary hyperlipidaemias are associated with
    A.   High-dose diuretic therapy
    B.   Some β-blockers
    C.   Corticosteroid therapy
    D.   Anorexia nervosa
    E.   Chronic renal failure

24. TFFFF

The ulnar nerve is derived from C7, C8 and T1. It is formed medial to the axillary artery. It does not give any branches in the upper arm. The ulnar nerve lies superficial to the flexor retinaculum and medial to the tendon of flexor carpi ulnaris.

25. FTTTF

Hepatitis B usually resolves completely. Problems only arise in the 10–20% of patients who become chronic carriers. Of these, 20% develop chronic hepatitis with its complications. The remaining 80% of carriers remain well but some eventually convert to hepatitis. Less than 0.5% of patients develop fulminant hepatic failure. Prophylaxis is by vaccination and immunoglobulin. Immunoglobulin is given for those with needle-stick injuries and to babies.

26. TTTTT

Endotracheal intubation disrupts cilial activity and permits bacterial leakage around the cuff of the endotracheal tube. Nasogastric tubes facilitate the retrograde spread of bacteria from the stomach. Increased length of stay increases the risk of development of nosocomial pulmonary infection. Increasing gastric pH leads to bacterial colonization of the stomach. Male gender has been reported to be a risk factor.

27. TTTTT

Lipid disorders are either primary or secondary. Secondary hyperlipidaemias are classified into hormonal causes (pregnancy, hypothyroidism, diabetes mellitus), nutritional factors (obesity, anorexia, alcohol), renal dysfunction (nephrotic syndrome, chronic renal failure), liver disease (primary biliary cirrhosis, extrahepatic obstruction), and iatrogenic (thiazides, β-blockers, steroids, sex hormone therapy and retinoids).

28. Concerning nitric oxide
   A.   Nitric oxide has neurotransmitter functions
   B.   Nitric oxide has a half-life of 90 s
   C.   Oxidative derivatives of nitric oxide are toxic
   D.   Inducible nitric oxide is found in hepatocytes
   E.   Inducible nitric oxide synthetase is dependent on intracellular calcium

29. The following increase the diffusion capacity for inspired carbon monoxide ($D_L CO$)
   A.   Chronic obstructive pulmonary disease
   B.   Congestive cardiac failure
   C.   Asthma
   D.   Anaemia
   E.   Perforated tympanic membrane

30. Inhaled prostacyclin
   A.   Causes vasodilatation by increasing intracellular cAMP levels
   B.   Is metabolized by red blood cells
   C.   Has a half-life of 2–3 min
   D.   Produces active metabolites
   E.   Has a beneficial effect on V/Q mismatch

28. **TFTTF**

Nitric oxide has neurotransmitter functions. It has a short half-life, in the order of 2–50 s. Oxidative derivatives of nitric oxide are toxic. Inducible nitric oxide synthetase found in macrophages and hepatocytes acts independently of intracellular calcium.

29. **FTTFT**

D_LCO is the rate of uptake of carbon monoxide per driving pressure of alveolar carbon monoxide. It is dependent on pulmonary vascular components, e.g. cardiac output, as well as membrane diffusing capacity. Interstitial lung and pulmonary vascular diseases decrease D_LCO. As carbon monoxide has a great affinity for haemoglobin, any disease that increases the relative amount of haemoglobin in the lung will increase D_LCO, e.g. congestive cardiac failure, asthma and diffuse pulmonary haemorrhage. A perforated ear drum may cause artifactually high D_LCO by allowing the escape of carbon monoxide by a non-pulmonary route.

30. **TFTFT**

Inhaled prostacyclin mediates vasodilatation by increasing intracellular cAMP levels. It undergoes spontaneous hydrolysis at physiological pH. It does not produce active metabolites. Inhaled prostacyclin has a half-life of 2–3 min. The vasodilator effect of inhaled prostacyclin is limited to pulmonary vessels perfusing ventilated areas. This has a beneficial effect on V/Q mismatch.

31. Concerning intra-arterial measurement of blood pressure
  A. Blood pressure is overestimated when the length of manometer tubing in a pressure transducer system is increased
  B. The oscillating frequency of the pressure transducer system should be <20 Hz in order to prevent amplification of the blood pressure signal
  C. Damping of the blood pressure signal occurs if the viscosity of the fluid in the pressure transducer system is increased
  D. A small air bubble in the manometer line causes overshoot of the pressure waveforms
  E. The diameter of the manometer tubing has no effect on the degree of damping of the blood pressure waveform

32. The symptoms and signs of hypokalaemia include
  A. Metabolic acidosis
  B. Increased renal concentrating capacity
  C. Diminished U waves on the electrocardiograph
  D. Prolonged QT interval on the electrocardiograph
  E. Ileus

33. Concerning the ITU management of acute pancreatitis
  A. Necrotizing pancreatitis has a mortality rate >60%
  B. CT scanning is superior to ultrasound in demonstrating biliary tract stones
  C. Infected necrotizing pancreatitis should be treated with antibiotics
  D. Serum lipase remains raised for longer than serum amylase
  E. Feeding should be commenced early via the enteral route

31. TFTFF

The natural frequency (fn) of a system is the frequency at which it resonates or 'rings'. Physiological frequencies similar to the natural frequency of the measuring system will be greatly amplified. Therefore, to prevent amplification, the natural frequency of the measuring system should be higher than the frequency of the physiological process it is measuring, which in the case of blood pressure is 20 Hz. Factors which reduce fn, e.g. increasing the length of manometer tubing, increasing the density of fluid in the tubing or reducing the diameter of tubing, will amplify the signal, causing the true blood pressure to be over-read. Factors that increase the degree of damping of the pressure signal are a reduction in manometer tubing diameter and increase in length, and an increase in viscosity and decrease in density of the fluid within the tubing. A small air bubble in the manometer line causes damping.

32. FFFFT

Hypokalaemia presents as muscle weakness, intestinal ileus, cardiac tachyarrhythmias, metabolic alkalosis, a decreased renal concentrating ability (polyuria, diminished glomerular filtration), myopathy, hypoventilation, myoglobinuria and characteristic electrocardiographic changes. These are initially sagging of the ST segment, T-wave depression and U-wave prominence. As the severity increases the T and U waves fuse. The PR interval is prolonged. The QT interval is normal.

33. FFFTF

Necrotizing pancreatitis has a mortality of 50%. CT scanning is inferior to ultrasound scanning when demonstrating biliary tract stones. Infected necrotizing pancreatitis is an indication for surgical debridement. Serum lipase remains raised for a longer period than amylase. Feeding should be commenced early; however, TPN is utilized to rest the gut.

34. Concerning vaporizers
    A.   Isoflurane will boil at room temperature (20°C) when the pressure is 0.5 atm
    B.   Vaporizers are made from metals with a low thermal conductivity, in order to prevent heat loss
    C.   At low flow rates (<250 ml/min) the output of variable bypass vaporizers is greater than the dial setting
    D.   Using the oxygen flush can result in higher vaporizer output concentration than the dialled setting
    E.   The boiling point of isoflurane is greater than that of enflurane

35. The Guedel stages of anaesthesia
    A.   Were originally observed in unpremedicated patients
    B.   Were originally observed in patients breathing ether and oxygen mixtures
    C.   At stage 3 plane I, the corneal reflex is depressed
    D.   At stage 3 plane III, breathing is diaphragmatic
    E.   Anal stretch may be uneventfully performed at stage 3 plane III

34. FFFTF

The boiling point is the temperature at which the vapour pressure equals atmospheric pressure. The boiling point of enflurane is 56.5°C. At 1 atmosphere the boiling point of isoflurane is 48.5°C whereas at 0.5 atmospheres it is 30°C. Vaporizers have a relatively high thermal conductivity to allow them to conduct heat from the atmosphere to the vapour chamber. The output of bypass type vaporizers is less than the dial setting at very low flow rates. This is because the pressure generated inside the vaporization chamber by the fresh gas is not enough to lift the volatile anaesthetic molecules towards the vaporizer outlet. At very high flow rates the output is less than the dial setting due to incomplete mixing of fresh gas and anaesthetic vapour. Use of the oxygen flush, as well as IPPV, causes back pressure within the vaporizer which, when released, allows vapour to escape back out through the inlet into the oncoming fresh gas. Part of this vapour containing fresh gas will then bypass the vaporizer chamber to be added to saturated carrier gas further downstream. This is known as the pumping effect.

35. FFFTF

The signs of anaesthesia described by Guedel were observed in patients premedicated with atropine and morphine, breathing ether and air mixtures. At stage 3 plane II the corneal reflex is depressed. At stage 3 plane III breathing is diaphragmatic. At stage 3 plane III anal stretch will cause laryngospasm.

36. Phaeochromocytoma
A. Falling haematocrit points towards adequate pre-operative preparation
B. Phenoxybenzamine is a competitive antagonist at α receptors
C. Propranolol is a useful first-line agent in the control of blood pressure
D. Droperidol is useful as a premedication
E. Neuroaxial blocks are useful in the control of intra-operative hypertension

37. The causes of secondary obesity include
A. Nifedipine
B. Ranitidine
C. Hyperparathyroidism
D. Carcinoid syndrome
E. Addison's disease

38. Tracheostomy
A. In paediatric tracheostomy a Bjork flap should be used
B. Paediatric tracheostomy should be at the level of the 1st and 2nd tracheal rings
C. The thyroid arteries are the arteries most commonly eroded by the tracheostomy tip
D. When performing the percutaneous approach, the tracheostomy should be sited inferior to the thyroid isthmus
E. Pneumothorax is a recognized complication

39. Following smoke inhalation
A. Plasma iron levels drop
B. Plasma copper levels increase
C. Pulmonary vascular pressure drops
D. Pulmonary oedema is of immediate onset
E. Lung compliance decreases

36. TFFFF
A dropping haematocrit indicates restoration of plasma volume. Phenoxybenzamine is a non-competitive antagonist forming covalent bonds with α receptors. Propranolol does not possess α-blocking activity. Administration to a patient who is not β-blocked can lead to severe hypertension. Droperidol has been reported to cause hypertension by release of catecholamines from the phaeochromocytoma. Neuroaxial block is ineffective as it is functioning at the preganglionic level, having no attenuation of the effect of circulating catecholamines.

37. FFFFF
Secondary obesity has many causes and it must be remembered that not all obesity is primary, i.e. dietary. Secondary obesity can be caused by hypothyroidism, Cushing's disease, insulin resistance, hypothalamic disorders, hypogonadism, and can be drug induced. Steroids are the obvious example of this. Between 80 and 90% of type II diabetics are obese. Questions are normally answered by a definition of diabetes and then the causes.

38. FFFFT
Paediatric tracheostomy should employ a longitudinal slit at the 2nd and 3rd tracheal rings. Arterial erosion by the tracheostomy tip most commonly involves the innominate artery. When utilizing the percutaneous approach the tracheostomy should be sited superior to the thyroid isthmus. Pneumothorax is a recognized complication.

39. TFFFT
Following the inhalation of smoke both plasma copper and iron levels drop within the first 48 h. Pulmonary vascular pressures rise. Subsequent pulmonary oedema arises during the following 2–3 days. Lung compliance decreases.

40. Regarding the Lambert–Eaton myasthenic syndrome
   A. The main clinical feature is fatigable muscle weakness
   B. Reflexes may show 'post-tetanic accentuation'
   C. The EMG is typical, with an increase in muscular response to repeated stimulation
   D. Sixty per cent of cases are associated with small (oat) cell carcinoma of the bronchus
   E. This autoimmune condition causes production of antibodies to presynaptic calcium channels, and this leads to reduced release of acetylcholine

41. The following drugs induce porphyria
   A. Thiopentone
   B. Propofol
   C. Flunitrazepam
   D. α-methyl dopa
   E. Droperidol

42. Regarding local anaesthetic blocks via the caudal route in children
   A. 0.5 ml/kg of 0.25% bupivacaine is required for hernia repair
   B. Neonates are at greater risk of anaesthetic toxicity than adults
   C. The maximum suggested volume of 0.25% bupivacaine is 30 ml
   D. 2 ml/kg of 0.25% bupivacaine is required for orchidopexy
   E. The maximum recommended dose of plain bupivacaine in children is 3 mg/kg

40. TTTTT
Similar in nature to myasthenia gravis in that it causes fatigable muscle weakness, the treatment and prognosis are different. Most are associated with lung malignancy, but it has been reported in other malignancies (stomach, prostate and breast). Occasionally it is not related to malignancy but is just autoimmune. Weakness may improve towards the end of the day and tendon reflexes are depressed or absent.

41. TFTTF
Porphyrias are a group of conditions in which one or more of the enzymes responsible for the synthesis of haem are defective, causing build-up of precursors in the haem pathway. Many of the drugs that precipitate an attack of porphyria are inducers of hepatic cytochrome P-450, which is the main consumer of haem in the liver. Induction of cytochrome P-450 therefore depletes the haem pool, with loss of negative feedback on aminolaevulinate (ALA) synthetase, the first enzyme in the synthesis of haem from succinyl CoA and glycine. This increases the rate of haem production and the build up of haem precursors in patients with porphyria. There are other questions on this subject in this book so you will be able to build up an extensive list of safe and unsafe drugs!

42. FTFFF
Armitage described volumes of caudally administered 0.25% bupivacaine to provide analgesia for procedures in children. Circumcision and hypospadias require 0.5 ml/kg while herniotomy and orchidopexy need 1 ml/kg. The maximum volume should not exceed 20 ml. Neonates are at increased risk of local anaesthetic toxicity because the half-lives are 2–3 times longer due to immature mycrosomal enzyme systems. In addition, there is reduced protein binding with an increase in free drug in the blood. The recommended safe dose for plain bupivacaine in children is 2 mg/kg.

43. During normal pregnancy
A. During uterine contraction, cardiac output can reach 15 l/min
B. The closing capacity of the lung increases during late pregnancy
C. MAC is reduced by approximately 40%
D. The concentration of all clotting factors increases by 10–50% by the third trimester
E. Tubular reabsorption of glucose during pregnancy is reduced

44. Gelofusine contains
A. 40 g/l of urea-linked gelatin
B. Less potassium per litre than haemaccel
C. Particles with an average molecular weight of 45 000
D. Less sodium per litre than haemaccel
E. 6.26 mmol/l of calcium

45. Anaesthesia and patients with sickle-cell disease
A. Tourniquets are absolutely contraindicated
B. Intra-operative transfusion of whole blood is preferable to packed cells
C. Pre-operative erythropoietin is useful
D. Cell-saving techniques in major surgery are useful
E. Elective surgery is absolutely contraindicated in the presence of acute infection

43. TFTFT

There is no significant change in closing capacity in pregnant women. However, FRC is reduced by 20% so that small airway closure occurs in 50% of supine mothers. The fall in MAC may be due, in part, to increased blood levels of progesterone, which can cause sedation. Fibrinogen and all clotting factors except V, IX and XIII increase by about 50% by term. Glycosuria is common due to the reduction in tubular glucose reabsorption.

44. FTFFF

A favourite MCQ. Learn the composition of all the fluids you give to patients. It may be boring, but is very useful for exam purposes. Gelofusine contains: 40 g/l succinylated gelatin, 154 mmol/l sodium, 125 mmol/l chloride, 0.4 mmol/l calcium and 0.4 mmol/l potassium. Haemaccel contains: 35 g/l urea-linked gelatin, 145 mmol/l sodium, 145 mmol/l chloride, 6.26 mmol/l calcium and 5.1 mmol/l potassium. The average molecular weight of both solutions is 35 000.

45. FTFFT

Tourniquets may be used successfully provided there is careful attention to exsanguination of the limb. Because of the increased levels of 2,3 DPG, whole blood transfusions are preferable to packed cell transfusions. Erythropoietin has not been shown to be useful. Cell-saving techniques are associated with sickling due to the cell-washing process. Elective surgery is absolutely contraindicated in the presence of infection, due to the increased risk of precipitating a crisis.

46. The following statements about the pulmonary artery catheter are true

A. When correctly wedged, pulmonary artery occlusion pressure is equal to pulmonary artery diastolic pressure

B. Left bundle branch block is a relative contraindication to insertion

C. Tricuspid stenosis is a relative contraindication to insertion

D. The incidence of major haemorrhage secondary to pulmonary artery rupture is up to 0.25%

E. Right ventricular ejection fraction may be calculated in certain circumstances

47. Regarding critical temperature and critical pressure

A. At room temperature, carbon dioxide is a gas

B. The critical pressure of oxygen is 50 bar

C. The critical temperature is the temperature at which a vapour cannot be liquefied whatever the pressure applied to it

D. The relationship between pressure and volume of an ideal gas at constant temperature is linear

E. The critical temperature of oxygen is $-183°C$

48. Regarding pregnancy-induced hypertension

A. The definition includes a single diastolic phase V $>110\,mmHg$

B. The definition includes two diastolic readings $>90\,mmHg$ which are 4 h apart after 20 weeks' pregnancy in a previously normotensive patient

C. A diastolic pressure $>90\,mmHg$ before 20 weeks suggests chronic hypertension

D. The definition includes proteinuria $>3\,g/day$

E. Eclampsia is defined as a generalized convulsion in pregnancy or labour or within 48 h of delivery

46. FTFTT
When correctly wedged the pulmonary artery diastolic pressure is greater than the pulmonary artery occlusion pressure. In the presence of left bundle branch block there is a 4% incidence of the pulmonary artery catheter causing right bundle branch block. This obviously leads to complete heart block. Tricuspid stenosis is an absolute contra-indication, its presence makes successful placement unlikely and if correctly placed the catheter will worsen the obstruction. Right ventricular ejection fraction may be measured using a pulmonary artery catheter with a rapid response thermistor.

47. FTFFF
The critical temperature is that above which a gas cannot be liquefied whatever the pressure applied to it. Above its critical temperature a substance is a gas, while below this temperature it is a vapour. As the critical temperature of carbon dioxide is 31°C, it is a vapour at room temperature. The critical temperature of oxygen is −118°C whereas its boiling point is −183°C. The pressure required to liquefy a vapour at the critical temperature is the critical pressure. The relationship between pressure and volume of an ideal gas at constant temperature (isotherm) is a rectangular hyperbola.

48. TTTFF
Eclampsia has a strict definition. It is a generalized convulsion in pregnancy, labour, or within 7 days after delivery, in the absence of epilepsy or another disorder predisposing to a convulsion. The 24-h urine collection should contain 0.3 g of protein. Questions that lead on from this are many. What are the pathophysiological changes? How is eclampsia managed? What are the complications of pre-eclampsia? How do you use magnesium in eclampsia?

49. Concerning paediatric cardiac surgery
- A. The degree of the stress response to cardiopulmonary bypass is similar to that in the adult
- B. Hypoglycaemia is a significant risk during surgery
- C. The prime volume represents a 100% increase in blood volume in infants
- D. The maximum duration of deep hypothermic circulatory arrest is 50–60 min
- E. Isolated regurgitant lesions are common in this age group

50. Inverse ratio ventilation
- A. Creates intrinsic PEEP
- B. The mean airway pressure remains unchanged
- C. Improves oxygenation in patients with ARDS
- D. Neuromuscular blockade is not required
- E. Has been used successfully in neonates

51. Concerning motor nerves
- A. Hip flexion is supplied by L2/L3
- B. Knee flexion is supplied by L5/S1
- C. Plantar flexion of the ankle is supplied by S1/S2
- D. Both adduction and abduction of the finger are supplied by T1
- E. Elbow flexion is supplied by C5/C6

52. Pneumoperitoneum is associated with
- A. Reduced pulmonary vascular resistance
- B. Increased systemic vascular resistance
- C. Increased transmural pressure across the heart
- D. Reduced cardiac output
- E. Reduced renal blood flow

49. FTFTF

As proportional exposure of the circulating volume to non-epithelialized surfaces is larger than in the adult, the extent of the stress response is greater. Hypoglycaemia is a major risk throughout the peri-operative period, especially with low output syndromes. In neonates and infants the prime volume represents an increase in blood volume of 200–300%. The maximum duration of deep hypothermic circulatory arrest is 50 to 60 min. Isolated regurgitant lesions are uncommon in paediatric practice.

50. TFTFT

Inverse ratio ventilation (IRV) produces an I:E ratio of greater than one. It produces intrinsic PEEP with an associated increase in mean airway pressures. It has been shown to improve oxygenation in ARDS. To facilitate IRV, deep levels of sedation are required and often neuromuscular blockade is needed. IRV was initially used successfully in neonates.

51. TTTTT

It is important to know all the sensory dermatomes and the motor myotomes for the exam as they are easy MCQ questions to score on. Look them up in any anatomy book.

52. FTFTT

Both systemic and pulmonary vascular resistance rise. As intrathoracic pressure rises secondary to the pneumoperitoneum, the transmural pressure across the heart drops. Both renal blood flow and glomerular filtration rate drop with the pneumoperitoneum.

53. The spinal cord and its blood supply
   A. The anterior and posterior spinal arteries have multiple anastomoses
   B. Occlusion of the anterior spinal artery leads to loss of proprioception
   C. The artery of Adamkiewicz arises from level L1–L4 in 80% of cases
   D. The anterior spinal artery is derived from the vertebral artery
   E. The anterior and posterior spinal arteries are paired

54. Regarding acute and chronic renal failure
   A. There is no bone disease in acute renal failure
   B. There is less pruritus in acute renal failure
   C. Chronic renal failure is defined as an abnormally low glomerular filtration rate of >6 months' duration
   D. Acute renal failure is defined as an abnormally low glomerular filtration rate of <6 months' duration
   E. Creatinine clearance decreases by approximately 1 ml/min/year from the age of 50 years

55. Tumour necrosis factor α
   A. Is an early mediator in the inflammatory response
   B. Is released from macrophages
   C. Is released from lymphocytes
   D. Is a phospholipid
   E. Inhibits arachidonic acid metabolism

53. FFFTF

The anterior and posterior spinal arteries do not anastomose with each other, hence occlusion of one of these vessels causes infarction of the cord. Occlusion of the anterior spinal artery causes loss of motor function and skin prick sensation with preservation of vibratory sense and proprioception. The artery of Adamkiewicz arises between levels T6–T9 in 60% of cases. The anterior spinal artery is derived from the vertebral artery. The posterior spinal artery is paired.

54. TTFFF

Acute renal failure is defined as an abnormally low glomerular filtration rate <3 months' duration. Similarly chronic renal failure is defined as an abnormally low glomerular filtration rate of >3 months' duration. The time in the definition is arbitrary but helps distinguish acute renal failure (usually reversible) from chronic renal failure (usually irreversible). Clinically it is not possible to distinguish between the two at presentation because the previous renal function is unknown. Creatinine clearance decreases by approximately 1 ml/min/year from the age of 35 years.

55. TTTFF

Tumour necrosis factor α is an early non-specific mediator in the inflammatory response. It is predominantly released from macrophages, but also from lymphocytes, natural killer cells and certain cells within the CNS. It is a polypeptide molecule which promotes the metabolism of arachidonic acid.

56. Regarding the mechanisms involved in pain perception
   A. Afferent pain nerves contain sympathetic fibres which increase the sensitivity of peripheral nociceptors
   B. The frequency of neuronal discharge in a nociceptic neurone remains constant if the stimulus remains constant
   C. Substance P is released from damaged tissue and sensitizes the nociceptive neurone to noradrenaline released by sympathetic nerves
   D. Aδ fibres primarily synapse in Rexed lamina I
   E. ATP released from damaged tissue stimulates nociceptive nerve endings

57. MRI scanning
   A. Non-metallic laryngoscopes may be used close to the magnetic field
   B. Pressure manometers retain their accuracy in the magnetic field
   C. Non-invasive blood pressure measurement does not cause problems
   D. ECG may disrupt the quality of the MRI picture
   E. Stainless steel is safe within the magnetic field

58. Regarding primary hyperaldosteronism
   A. It causes hypertension due to excess of the mineralocorticoid aldosterone
   B. It is normally caused by an adrenal carcinoma
   C. It causes hyperkalaemic hypertension
   D. Hypokalaemia suppresses aldosterone production even in those with tumours
   E. It is the most common endocrine cause of hypertension

56. TFFTT

Nociceptive neurones exhibit plasticity, which means that the frequency of discharge varies to a constant stimulus, i.e. the nerves become more sensitive. Substance P is released from free nerve endings of afferent pain fibres in response to trauma. It causes local vasodilatation and increases vascular permeability that causes local inflammation. It also stimulates the release of interleukins and arachidonic acid, which further sensitizes pain afferents. Potassium, hydrogen ions, 5-HT, interleukins and prostaglandins as well as ATP stimulate nociceptive nerve endings.

57. FFTTT

Non-metallic laryngoscopes may not be used as the batteries within are influenced by the magnetic field. Pressure manometers do not work in the presence of the magnetic field. Non-invasive blood pressure measurement is used successfully. Wires from the ECG may pick up stray radiofrequency signals distorting the MRI image. Stainless steel is not attracted to the magnetic field.

58. TFFTT

Primary hyperaldosteronism is so named because it is necessary to distinguish it from disorders which have a high level of aldosterone secondary to other causes such as accelerated hypertension or renal artery stenosis. The causes of primary hyperaldosteronism are benign adrenal tumour (most common), bilateral adrenal hyperplasia, adrenal carcinoma (rare) and pseudoprimary hyperaldosteronism (liquorice ingestion). Hypokalaemic hypertension occurs. Hypokalaemia suppresses aldosterone production and must be corrected before hormone levels are taken.

59. **Inotropic agents**
    A. Glucagon increases myocardial contractility
    B. Dobutamine acts primarily upon β_2 receptors
    C. Dobutamine is devoid of α activity
    D. Isoprenaline raises pulmonary artery occlusion pressure
    E. Isoprenaline is associated with oliguria

60. **Concerning the ankle block**
    A. The saphenous nerve is subcutaneous at the level of the ankle
    B. The sural nerve supplies the medial aspect of the foot
    C. The tibial nerve supplies the plantar surface of the lateral 3 toes
    D. The deep peroneal nerve innervates the contiguous areas of the 1st and 2nd toes
    E. The superficial peroneal nerve may be blocked immediately anterior to the medial malleolus

61. **The following tests of coagulation relate solely to the intrinsic coagulation pathway**
    A. Activated clotting time
    B. Prothrombin time
    C. Reptilase time
    D. Thrombin time
    E. Bleeding time

62. **Regarding pulse oximetry**
    A. Carboxyhaemoglobin results in an overestimation of the oxygen saturation of haemoglobin
    B. Methaemoglobin results in an underestimation of the oxygen saturation of haemoglobin
    C. One of the isobestic points of oxyhaemoglobin and deoxyhaemoglobin is 805 nm
    D. The light sources used by pulse oximeters are dichromatic light-emitting diodes
    E. Pulse oximeters reflect P_aO_2 more accurately at levels above 11 kPa

59. TFFFT

Glucagon increases myocardial contractility via increases in cAMP. Dobutamine acts primarily on β_1 receptors with modest effects on the α_1 receptor. Isoprenaline lowers pulmonary artery occlusion pressure. It may cause oliguria by dilatation of muscle vasculature, diverting blood away from vital organs.

60. TFFTF

The saphenous nerve becomes subcutaneous at the lateral side of the knee joint. The sural nerve supplies the lateral aspect of the foot. Terminal branches of the tibial nerve supply the plantar aspect of all the toes. The deep peroneal nerve supplies the contiguous areas of the 1st and 2nd toes. The superficial peroneal nerve may be blocked above and medial to the lateral malleolus.

61. TFFFF

Clotting is difficult to understand but is easy to write MCQs about. This is a bad combination! Thrombin and reptilase time measure the common pathway, while the extrinsic pathway is monitored using the prothrombin time and INR. Partial thromboplastin time, activated clotting time and activated partial thromboplastin time measure the intrinsic pathway.

62. TTTFF

The pulse oximeter emits light from monochromatic diodes, one with a wavelength of 660 nm and the other with a wavelength of 940 nm. Carboxyhaemoglobin has a similar absorbance to oxyhaemoglobin at 660 nm and results in an overestimation of the true oxygen saturation. Methaemoglobin mimics deoxyhaemoglobin at 660 nm and its presence drops the true oxygen saturation reading to about 85%. Due to the shape of the oxygen dissociation curve, oxygen saturation more accurately reflects P_aO_2 when this is less than 11 kPa (steep part of curve) compared to above 11 kPa (flat part of the curve).

63. The following factors have proven effects on the distribution of local anaesthetic following subarachnoid injection
- A. Barbotage
- B. Patient height
- C. Rate of injection
- D. Direction of the bevel on injection
- E. Position of the patient immediately after injection

64. The causes of aseptic meningitis include
- A. Enteroviruses
- B. Mumps virus
- C. Tuberculosis
- D. Leptospirosis
- E. Cryptococcus

65. Metabolic alkalosis occurs in the following conditions
- A. Hyperventilation
- B. Potassium deficiency
- C. Hyperaldosteronism
- D. Aspirin poisoning
- E. Erysipelas

66. In the management of oesophageal varices
- A. A Sengstaken–Blakemore tube should be left in situ for a maximum of 12 h
- B. Rebleeding is rare after removal of the Sengstaken–Blakemore tube
- C. Endoscopic sclerotherapy controls bleeding in 90% of cases
- D. Vasopressin may be safely used in patients with coronary artery disease
- E. Somatostatin has a longer duration of action than octreotide

63. FTFFT

Only patient height and position immediately after injection have been shown to have effects on the distribution of local anaesthetic following subarachnoid injection.

64. TTTTT

Aseptic meningitis is more common in the summer and in boys. It is characterized by lymphocytes in the cerebrospinal fluid. Partially treated bacterial meningitis should also be included in addition to the list included in the question. Viral aseptic meningitis is usually self-limiting and complete recovery is expected within a few days of the disease onset.

65. FTTFF

Erysipelas is infection of the deep dermis and subcutis in which lymphadenitis occurs. It is not relevant to the question! Don't guess! Hyperventilation causes a respiratory alkalosis. The causes of a metabolic alkalosis include pre-renal causes such as extra-renal loss of acid (vomiting, nasogastric suction, congenital alkalosis) and ingestion of alkali (sodium bicarbonate as an alkali). The renal causes are deficiencies interfering with tubular dysfunction (potassium deficiency, hypovolaemia), and other causes of renal dysfunction (hyperaldosteronism, diuretics). Finally, iatrogenic causes such as over-correction of an acidosis exist. Potassium deficiency leads to hydrogen ion wasting as it is preferentially absorbed.

66. FFTFF

The Sengstaken–Blakemore tube should only remain in situ for 24 h to reduce the danger of oesophageal rupture. Re-bleeding after removal is common. Endoscopic sclerotherapy successfully controls haemorrhage in 90%. Vasopressin should be avoided in patients with coronary artery disease because of its coronary vasoconstrictor properties. Octreotide is a long-acting analogue of somatostatin.

67. **Regarding the electroencephalogram (EEG) and components derived from it**
    A. β waves have a higher amplitude and a lower frequency than δ waves
    B. The spectral edge frequency is the EEG frequency below which 95% activity is present
    C. The amplitude of the auditory evoked response (AER) waveform is reduced by increasing concentrations of inhalational anaesthetics
    D. The amplitude of EEG waves is measured in millivolts (mV)
    E. The frequency of EEG waves is reduced with increasing depth of anaesthesia

68. **The following are side effects of lithium**
    A. Agranulocytosis
    B. Hypernatraemia
    C. Abdominal pain
    D. Goitre
    E. Diabetes insipidus

69. **Regarding chickenpox**
    A. Varicella-zoster virus is the herpes group virus responsible for it
    B. The virus can remain dormant in the motor ganglion for many years
    C. The thorax is the most commonly affected part of the body in shingles
    D. The ophthalmic division of the trigeminal nerve is the most commonly affected
    E. Post-herpetic neuralgia in the young is normally a result of immuno-compromise

67. FTTFT

β waves have a high frequency and low amplitude. The frequency decreases and the amplitude increases through waves α and θ, to δ. The frequency of the EEG falls with increasing depth of anaesthesia. The spectral edge indicates the overall frequencies present in the EEG. Therefore, the lower the spectral edge frequency, the deeper the level of anaesthesia. The amplitude of the AER reflects anaesthetic depth, falling with increasing concentrations of inhalational and intravenous anaesthetics and rising in response to surgical stimulation. The amplitude of the EEG and its variables is measured in microvolts (μV).

68. FFTTT

Lithium has a narrow therapeutic index. Symptoms of mild toxicity include nausea, vomiting, abdominal pain, diarrhoea, sedation and tremor. At higher plasma concentrations lithium causes hyperreflexia, confusion, fits, coma and cardiac arrhythmias. Goitre occurs due to an inhibition of the production of thyroxine. Hypothyroidism rarely occurs. Lithium inhibits the action of antidiuretic hormone on the kidneys producing a nephrogenic diabetes insipidus. The ECG may show T-wave depression and widening of the QRS complex. The number of neutrophils may also be increased.

69. TTTTT

Varicella-zoster is a DNA virus. Reactivation after chickenpox occurs as immunity wanes with age or following immunosuppression. Acyclovir given at the time of the shingles attack may decrease post-herpetic neuralgia. Post-herpetic neuralgia is a subject that must be known because it is frequently seen in chronic pain clinics, and treatment, as in all chronic pain, is directed towards empathy, drugs, nerve blocks, complementary techniques and regular follow-up.

70. Cholinergic crisis in myasthenia gravis
  A.   The condition is improved by edrophonium
       administration
  B.   Respiratory difficulty is not a feature
  C.   Abdominal cramps are a feature
  D.   Constipation is a feature
  E.   Bulbar palsy may ensue

71. Regarding intra-ocular pressure
  A.   The normal intra-ocular pressure is 10–20 mmHg
  B.   Etomidate increases intra-ocular pressure
  C.   Calcium channel blockers reduce intra-ocular pressure
  D.   Pre-operative acetazolamide reduces the rise in intra-
       ocular pressure associated with suxamethonium
  E.   Competitive neuromuscular blocking drugs have no
       effect on intra-ocular pressure

72. Regarding neonatal physiology
  A.   Glomerular filtration rate (GFR) reaches adult values
       by the third month
  B.   Hyponatraemia is more common in neonates than in
       adults
  C.   The normal haemoglobin concentration in a neonate is
       17.0–22.0 g/dl
  D.   The normal neonatal blood volume is 80 ml/kg
  E.   The neonatal head contributes 21% to the total body
       surface area

73. Hypocalcaemia is caused by
  A.   Massive citrated blood transfusion
  B.   Phenytoin therapy
  C.   Thyrotoxicosis
  D.   Acute renal failure
  E.   Pancreatitis

70. FFTFT

A cholinergic crisis in myasthenia gravis is diagnosed by worsening of the condition with edrophonium. Excessive secretions may exacerbate respiratory difficulty. Abdominal symptoms include cramps and diarrhoea. A cholinergic crisis may lead to a bulbar palsy.

71. TFFTF

Apart from ketamine that increases it, all the other intravenous and inhalational anaesthetic drugs reduce intra-ocular pressure. Acetazolamide reduces intra-ocular pressure by blocking the formation of aqueous humour, while calcium channel blockers have no effect. Non-depolarizing muscle relaxants reduce intra-ocular pressure by decreasing tone in the extra-ocular muscles.

72. FTTTT

GFR at birth is 20–25 ml/min. It increases to 35–50 ml/min by the end of the first week and to 55–60 ml/min by the third month. Hyponatraemia is more likely in neonates as they have a relatively short loop of Henle which decreases the ability of the kidney to retain sodium via the ascending limb. In a neonate the head comprises 21% of the total body surface area whereas in an adult it is only 9%.

73. TTFFT

The causes of hypocalcaemia can be classified into three categories. Firstly those that are vitamin D dependent, and these include vitamin D deficiency or malabsorption and impaired vitamin D metabolism (chronic renal failure, chronic liver failure, phenytoin and congenital). Secondly there is hypoparathyroidism or parathormone resistance and this includes post-operative parathyroidectomy, idiopathic, infiltrative (haemochromatosis), neonatal and hypomagnesaemia. Thirdly there is a miscellaneous group that includes phosphate therapy, pancreatitis, massive citrated blood transfusion, and acute rhabdomyolysis.

74. In an acute severe asthma attack
- A.   Lung elastic recoil increases
- B.   Functional residual capacity (FRC) increases
- C.   Total lung capacity (TLC) increases
- D.   Intrinsic PEEP is present
- E.   Pulmonary vascular resistance increases

75. Phosphodiesterase inhibitors
- A.   Produce peripheral vasodilatation
- B.   Reduce preload and afterload
- C.   Myocardial oxygen consumption is increased
- D.   Prevent the breakdown of cAMP
- E.   Milrinone is a phosphodiesterase II inhibitor

76. Signs and symptoms of acute water intoxication include
- A.   Blurred vision
- B.   Transient blindness
- C.   Hypotension
- D.   Hypertension
- E.   Diarrhoea

77. Ketamine
- A.   Has active metabolites
- B.   Is presented as a racemic mixture
- C. $t_{1/2\alpha}$ is 3–5 min
- D.   Enflurane reduces ketamine clearance
- E.   Raises intracranial pressure

74. FTTTT

During an acute severe asthma attack lung elastic recoil is reduced. Air trapping causes a raised FRC and TLC. At the end of expiration alveolar pressure remains positive. This is intrinsic PEEP. Pulmonary vascular resistance rises secondary to increased intra-thoracic pressure.

75. TTFTF

The phosphodiesterase III inhibitors increase the force of myocardial contraction as well as relaxing vascular smooth muscle. Thus both preload and afterload are reduced. Myocardial oxygen consumption is not increased. Phosphodiesterase III inhibitors prevent the destruction of cAMP. Milrinone is a phosphodiesterase III inhibitor.

76. TTTTF

Acute water intoxication occurs as a result of irrigating fluid absorption most commonly in transurethral resection of the prostate. Signs and symptoms occur most obviously when the serum sodium falls below 120 mmol/l. Regional anaesthesia allows for an early diagnosis, and vomiting is often the first sign of toxicity. Any sign or symptom can occur but those most likely are vomiting, confusion, restlessness, blurred vision, transient blindness, convulsions, bradycardia, asystole, hypotension, hypertension and pulmonary oedema.

77. TTFTT

Norketamine has 20–30% of the activity of ketamine. Ketamine is presented as a racemic mixture. The $t_{1/2\alpha}$ of ketamine is 11–16 min. As clearance of ketamine is equivalent to liver blood flow, any drug that reduces liver blood flow will reduce ketamine clearance. Ketamine uniquely among the induction agents raises intracranial pressure.

78. The management of a patient with anaphylaxis at induction of anaesthesia includes
  A.   10 ml of calcium gluconate
  B.   Sodium bicarbonate should be given immediately
  C.   0.5–1 ml of 1:1000 adrenaline intravenously
  D.   100–300 mg of hydrocortisone intravenously
  E. H_2 antagonists can be useful

79. Coeliac plexus block
  A.   Preganglionic sympathetic fibres from T5–T12 relay in the coeliac ganglia
  B.   The coeliac plexus lies between the first and second lumbar vertebrae
  C.   Coeliac plexus block is used to treat the pain of chronic pancreatitis
  D.   Ablation of the coeliac plexus results in impotence
  E.   Dural tap is a complication

80. Regarding intracranial pressure (ICP)
  A.   The normal ICP is 2–4 kPa
  B.   ICP is most accurately measured using a subdural catheter
  C.   The intracranial pressure–volume relationship is determined by injecting 1 ml of normal saline into the lateral ventricle
  D.   Cerebral perfusion pressure is normally 50 mmHg
  E.   Lundberg's C-waves are not pathological

81. Regarding the trace elements
  A.   Zinc deficiency increases the risk of infection
  B.   Copper deficiency causes a refractory anaemia
  C.   Chronic manganese intoxication causes lung fibrosis
  D.   Zinc requirements are increased in high gastrointestinal output states
  E.   Taurine deficiency prolongs the effects of sedation in ITU patients

78. FFFTT

The Association of Anaesthetists have guidelines on this and it is essential to know them. Calcium is not required. Sodium bicarbonate is given as guided by blood gases only. The doses of adrenaline are 0.5–1 ml of 1:10 000 IV and 0.5–1 ml of 1:1000 subcutaneously. Slow IV chlorpheniramine, 10–20 mg, can also be given.

79. TFTTT

The coeliac plexus lies between T12 and L1. More commonly coeliac plexus block is used to relieve malignant pain. Penetration of the intervertebral foramen can lead to dural puncture. Other complications include damage to the great vessels, aortoduodenal fistula and hypotension.

80. FFTFF

The normal ICP is 0.6–1.3 kPa (5–10 mmHg). It is most accurately measured using a catheter inserted into the lateral ventricle. The intracranial pressure–volume relationship is determined by injecting 1 ml of normal saline into the lateral ventricle and measuring the change in pressure. Cerebral perfusion pressure (CPP) is normally 80 mmHg. If CPP falls to 50 mmHg signs of cerebral ischaemia appear. C-waves have a frequency of 6/min and are related to cyclical changes in arterial pressure in the presence of cerebral disorders.

81. TTFTF

Zinc deficiency also causes delayed wound healing, diarrhoea, alopecia and a scaly rash. Zinc requirements are increased in diarrhoea and high-output fistulae. Chronic manganese ingestion causes a Parkinsonian-like illness. Taurine causes reversible retinal dysfunction in children.

82. Lactic acid
A.   Lactic acid is formed by glycolysis
B.   Lactic acidosis is caused by alcohol consumption
C.   Lactic acid levels in a stored sample of blood fall with time
D.   Cyanide poisoning causes an acidosis with a normal or reduced lactate level due to a reduction in cellular carbohydrate metabolism
E.   Lactic acidosis causes an anion gap metabolic acidosis

83. Regarding the syndrome of inappropriate anti-diuretic hormone release (SIADH)
A.   It is associated with hypovolaemia
B.   Plasma osmolality is usually <280 mosmol/kg and the urine osmolality is >75 mosmol/kg
C.   It is caused by pulmonary tuberculosis
D.   Primary therapy involves hypertonic saline
E.   DDAVP is useful in the treatment of resistant cases

84. Anaesthesia for carotid endarterectomy
A.   Superficial cervical plexus block is performed by subcutaneous infiltration of local anaesthetic along the anterior border of the posterior belly of sternomastoid
B.   Deep cervical plexus block anaesthetizes C3–C5
C.   Shallow breathing is associated with deep cervical plexus block
D.   The hypoglossal nerve can be blocked
E.   Stump pressures correlate closely with neurological status in the awake patient undergoing carotid endarterectomy following carotid cross clamping

82. TTFFT

Lactic acid is formed from the anaerobic metabolism of carbohydrates. Causes include: hypoxia, hypoperfusion, sepsis, diabetic ketoacidosis, liver disease, cyanide poisoning and alcohol. Lactic acid levels in stored blood rise as the cells continually metabolize glucose to lactate. The anion gap = [Na] − ([Cl] + [HCO$_3$]). Lactic acid is titrated by bicarbonate. Therefore, lactic acidosis causes a rise in the anion gap as bicarbonate is used up, hence the term anion gap metabolic acidosis.

83. FFTFF

To diagnose SIADH the patient must be normovolaemic or hypervolaemic, the urine must be inappropriately concentrated (>100 mosmol/kg), and renal, cardiac, hepatic, adrenal and thyroid function must be normal. Causes include raised intracranial pressure, cerebral trauma, tumour, infection and haemorrahge, and pulmonary conditions such as TB, pneumonia, asthma, IPPV and bronchiectasis. Malignancies may produce ADH-like substances. First-line treatment is water restriction. DDAVP, which has an ADH-like action, is used to treat diabetes insipidus.

84. FFTTF

Superficial cervical plexus block is performed by subcutaneous infiltration of local anaesthetic along the posterior border of the posterior belly of sternomastoid. C2 to C4 are blocked with deep cervical plexus block. Complications of this type of block include phrenic and recurrent laryngeal nerve block, seizures from intra-arterial injection and total spinal or epidural block. Stump pressures do not accurately reflect neurological status during carotid cross clamping in the awake patient.

85. **Regarding diathermy**
    A. Bipolar diathermy requires a patient plate
    B. The current frequency used by diathermy is 0.5–1 kHz
    C. The risk of patient electrocution is reduced by earthing the diathermy
    D. Sensing pacemakers are more likely to be interfered with than demand pacemakers
    E. Unipolar diathermy causes less pacemaker interference than bipolar diathermy

86. **Regarding cardiac electromechanical dissociation (EMD)**
    A. Hypothermia is a cause
    B. Calcium chloride is useful in β-blocker-induced EMD
    C. Glucagon is a cause
    D. It can be caused by tricyclic antidepressant overdose
    E. It can be caused by digoxin overdose

87. **Concerning statistics**
    A. The statistical power of a study is the probability of achieving the same result if the experiment was repeated
    B. Type I error occurs when an experiment finds a difference between study groups when in fact no difference exists
    C. The t-test compares the means of two groups
    D. The Mann–Whitney test compares nominal or categorical data in two groups
    E. An experiment returning a 'p' value of <0.02 would be termed not significant

85. FFFTF

With unipolar diathermy the forceps act as one electrode and the patient plate acts as another, while with bipolar diathermy current passes through the tissues from one limb of the forceps to the other and no patient plate is required. Bipolar diathermy causes less pacemaker interference. The frequency of the electrical current used in surgical diathermy is 0.5–1 MHz. If the patient plate is earthed, current may take another route to earth, e.g. through a metal drip stand, which the patient may be touching, leading to electrocution. Therefore, the diathermy is isolated from earth so that stray current can no longer flow through the patient to earth.

86. TTFTT

The causes of EMD are hypovolaemia, hypoxia, hypothermia, tension pneumothorax, cardiac tamponade, massive PE, acidosis and myocardial infarction. Drug overdosage with tricyclic antidepressants, digoxin, β-blockers and calcium channel blockers also cause EMD. Glucagon treats EMD secondary to β-blockers.

87. FTTTF

Statistical power is the ability to detect an effect when one is present. Type I error in other words is a false positive error. A type II error unsurprisingly is when a false negative result occurs. When data are non-numerical, e.g. gender (male/female), mathematical operations are not valid. In these cases tests of significance such as the t-test or analysis of variance will not work. The Mann–Whitney and Chi squared tests are examples of tests which can be used in these circumstances. Usually in medical papers $p < 0.05$ is considered to be the upper limit of statistical significance.

88. The following are useful in treating myoglobinuria
   A.   Fresh frozen plasma (FFP)
   B.   Thiazide diuretics
   C.   Mannitol
   D.   Bicarbonate
   E.   Copper

89. Diuretics
   A.   Ethacrynic acid is a loop diuretic
   B.   Triamterine acts on the proximal convoluted tubule
   C.   Spironolactone is a non-competitive aldosterone
        inhibitor
   D.   Frusemide inhibits chloride reabsorption at the thick
        ascending loop of Henle
   E.   Acetazolamide acts at the distal convoluted tubule

**90. The following are clinical findings in a patient with digoxin
   toxicity**
   A.   Abdominal pain
   B.   Lymphocytosis
   C.   Complete heart block
   D.   Hypomagnesaemia
   E.   Paraesthesiae

88. TFTTF

FFP contains haptoglobulin which binds free haemoglobin and may protect renal function. Vigorous fluid therapy and maintenance of renal blood flow and urine output with osmotic diuretics, as well as alkalinization of the urine with bicarbonate, are useful.

89. TFFTF

There are five types of diuretic:
(1) Carbonic anhydrase inhibitors, e.g. acetazolamide, which act on the proximal convoluted tubule.
(2) Thiazides, e.g. bendrofluazide, which act on the cortical diluting segment just proximal to the distal convoluted tubule.
(3) Potassium-sparing diuretics, e.g. spironolactone and triamterine, which competitively inhibit aldosterone in the distal convoluted tubule.
(4) Loop diuretics, e.g. furosemide (new name), bumetanide and ethacrynic acid, which inhibit chloride reabsorption at the thick ascending loop of Henle.
(5) Osmotic diuretics, e.g. mannitol and urea.

90. TFTFT

Digoxin toxicity causes anorexia, nausea, vomiting, abdominal pain, confusion, paraesthesia and amblyopia. ECG changes are non-specific and include premature ventricular contractions, bigeminy, delayed A–V node conduction and heart block. Hypomagnesaemia as well as hypokalaemia, hypercalcaemia, advanced age and hypothyroidism predispose to digoxin toxicity.

91. Regarding Arsenal Football Club (AFC)
    A.   Arsenal won the famed double of League and FA Cup
         in 1971/2
    B.   We support Arsenal
    C.   Arsenal are boring
    D.   Arsenal invariably win one-nil
    E.   Arsenal is life, the rest is just detail

91. FFFFT

Arsenal won the double in 1970/71 when they beat Liverpool
in the FA Cup Final at Wembley in extra time with a Charlie
George goal. They had won the league a few days earlier.
Arsenal won the double more recently in 1997/98, winning
the league with two games to spare on a glorious May day at
The Home of Football (Highbury). On that most wonderful
of days Arsenal scored four outstanding goals against
Everton. They went on to win the FA Cup against
Newcastle. Although the life of one of the authors is devoted
to Arsenal, of the other two, one is not interested in
football!, while the other, for reasons known only to himself,
supports Preston North End (although he supports Arsenal
in the real world). Arsenal are not boring and often win in
great style, scoring many unforgettable goals. Questions C
and D, therefore, were put in to give you easy marks!
ARSENAL IS LIFE, THE REST IS JUST DETAIL!

Index

Vacuum systems, 228
Van Slyke apparatus, 36
Vancomycin, 46
Vanillyl mandelic acid, 12
Vaporizer in circle, 104
Vaporizers, 132, 180, 194, 258
Vapour pressure, 94
Vapours, *see* Gases
Varicella-zoster, 278
Velosulin, 60
Venous pressure, 28
Ventilation, 172, 224
  inverse ratio, 268
  positive pressure, 32
  systems, 32, 104, 212, 224

weaning from, 70
Viscosity, 194
Volts, 76
Vomiting, 122

Water intoxication, 282
Wavelengths, 12
Weaning from ventilation, 70
Weight, 210, *see also* Obesity
White tube, 132

Zeolites, 228
Zinc, 284